Research Methods for Therapists

Research Methods for Therapists

Avril Drummond

The Medical School,
University of Nottingham

Consultant editor:
Jo Campling

CHAPMAN & HALL

London · Weinheim · New York · Tokyo · Melbourne · Madras

Published by Chapman & Hall, 2–6 Boundary Row, London SE1 8HN, UK

Chapman & Hall, 2–6 Boundary Row, London SE1 8HN, UK

Chapman & Hall GmbH, Pappelallee 3, 69469 Weinheim, Germany

Chapman & Hall USA, 115 Fifth Avenue, New York NY 10003, USA

Chapman & Hall Japan, ITP-Japan, Kyowa Building, 3F, 2-2-1 Hira-kawacho, Chiyoda-ku, Tokyo 102, Japan

Chapman & Hall Australia, 102 Dodds Street, South Melbourne, Victoria 3205, Australia

Chapman & Hall India, R. Seshadri, 32 Second Main Road, CIT East, Madras 600 035, India

Distributed in the USA and Canada by Singular Publishing Group Inc., 4284 41st Street, San Diego, California 92105

First edition 1996

© 1996 Avril Drummond

Typeset in 10/12 Times by Cambrian Typesetters, Frimley, Surrey

Printed in Great Britain by Hartnolls Ltd. Bodmin

ISBN 0 412 45950 7   1 56593 207 2 (USA)

A catalogue record for this book is available from the British Library

Library of Congress Catalog Card Number: 96–083981

∞ Printed on permanent acid-free text paper, manufactured in accordance with ANSI/NISO Z39.48-1992 and ANSI/NISO Z39.48-1984 (Permanence of Paper).

For my Mum and Dad

Contents

Preface

This book is aimed at beginners. If you are totally confused and dismayed at the prospect of undertaking a research project, read on. If you are an expert in research, this is not the book for you unless you merely wish to revise your existing knowledge.

Above all this book is intended as an outline and a guide. It does not provide a definitive recipe on how to conduct a research project. You will learn by your own studies which methods and techniques suit you best and how to modify ideas to meet your own requirements.

NB

Therapist is referred to as *she* in the text for simplicity.

Acknowledgements

I owe particular thanks to Dr Naomi Fraser-Holland for her substantial contributions to the production of this book. My sincere thanks also go to Marion Walker, Dr John Gladman, Dr Nadina Lincoln, Dr Alison Hammond and Julia Nuthall for ideas, information and advice, and to Jane Greaves for her wonderful cartoons. I would also like to acknowledge the assistance of colleagues at the Stroke Research Unit, City Hospital, Nottingham, and at the Derby School of Occupational Therapy. I am grateful to Jo Campling for her support and guidance and to the staff at Chapman & Hall for all their assistance. Finally special thanks to my husband, Dr Tim Daniel, for his encouragement and good humour.

Avril Drummond
December 1995

Introduction

DEFINITION OF RESEARCH

What is research? How would you describe it to someone who wants to become a therapist? Let us look at some definitions of research to see whether they would help you answer these questions.

The *Oxford Dictionary* defines research as a 'course of critical study' while Mosby's *Medical and Nursing Dictionary* says that it is 'diligent inquiry or examination of data, reports and observations in search of facts and principles'. Calnan (1984) describes research as 'the making of observations, proposing a hypothesis to explain them, testing the hypothesis by experiment, and reaching a conclusion'. The scope of these definitions increases from the first to the third but together they cover the general characteristics of research. After you have read this book, you may feel that you can make a thorough job of telling a novice just what research has to offer.

What makes a good researcher? According to Hockey (1985) the successful researcher has five attributes:

- curiosity
- competence
- integrity
- common sense
- a sense of humour.

It would be just as appropriate to list these attributes for the successful therapist who can rightfully claim all five. So how does a successful therapist become a successful researcher? Basically, by exploring what is written about the research process, working with research colleagues and practising what they and the textbooks advise. As you read, you are already on your way.

> Research should not be an elevated and highly technical business conducted by academics in isolation from the world.
>
> Reid and Boore (1987: 6)

Research and therapy

Many therapists view research with some suspicion. They feel that it is not included in the job description of a 'real' therapist. They see their role only as practitioners of their profession and view research as unrelated. However, this is unreasonable: all therapists are essentially researchers by the very nature of their work. The basic tools of the researcher are the basic tools of any therapist. Consider the following examples.

If a therapist is referred a patient with a diagnosis of which she has no experience, what does she do? Probably she discusses the diagnosis with her colleagues, with someone she thinks may be an expert in this field, or she looks for some literature which will provide her with the answers she needs in order to plan a treatment programme.

A therapist notices that a patient responds better to therapy in a particular setting or at a particular time of day. This prompts her to rearrange the treatment programme to make the best use of the favourable conditions she has observed.

If one group of patients who have nerve lesions and are receiving one sort of treatment seem to do better than another group who have similar problems but are being given different treatment, the therapist will try using the first treatment on both groups.

These are all examples of using the principles of research in day-to-day practice. Questions constantly emerge from clinical practice and research is the way in which we find logical answers. The therapist already has the basic skills of research: observation, looking for answers to questions, testing ideas and adjusting treatment plans where evidence supports a fresh approach. Only modification of these skills is necessary to promote the more structured investigation known as research.

Research as part of practice is essential, not only for the wellbeing of our patients and clients, but for the survival of the therapeutic professions. Today there is great emphasis on value for money. Thus it is vital to demonstrate that our treatments work and are delivered in the most cost-effective way. The paramedical professions need a solid foundation based on more than tradition or ideas borrowed and applied from other disciplines. Research is needed to test theory and practice in the therapeutic professions. In this way a sound knowledge base can be developed. It is no longer good enough to say that we know something works, we must provide evidence that it does. Research can no longer be dismissed as a luxury. It must be accepted as a necessary part of providing the quality of care our patients and clients deserve.

WHY DO RESEARCH?

There are many reasons, professional and personal, why therapists decide
to begin research projects. Among these, the most common are:

1. As a course requirement. The majority of undergraduate and postgraduate courses now stipulate that students must carry out a research
   project.
2. To produce material for publication.
3. To improve prospects for promotion.
4. To specialize and gain expertise in an area.
5. To gather information that can be used to plead a case of need, for
   example to the health authority for more staff.
6. To take up the challenge of unravelling an interesting problem.

Research can assist in the development of an enquiring attitude in all
aspects of work. It is important in helping therapists to evaluate the work
of others in a critical and constructive way. In summary, there is no
substitute for research in the survival of the professions.

The research process: descriptions and the real thing

It is important that the therapist approaching the field of investigation
realizes from the beginning that the research process is much more fluid
than it appears on paper. Consequently, although the chapters of this book
are laid out rather like a cookery recipe, in that all the stages of the
research process are explained individually and in a particular order, this is
only for ease of understanding. Many of the factors discussed separately
really occur simultaneously and not in such a regimented sequence.

Consider, for example, the format of the first chapter. This deals first
with thinking of a research idea, then with talking it over with colleagues
and finally with carrying out the literature search. However, this format
merely simplifies the situation. In reality the idea may be established from
talking to colleagues or the literature search may be conducted at the same
time as the idea is being brought into shape. Similarly, Chapter 6 deals with
writing-up the research. This suggests that writing-up is done when the
whole project is completed. Although many researchers prefer to work in
this way, others prefer to write-up as they go along. Consequently you
must use the information in this book in the way that suits your needs. This
is best done by attempting to overview the whole research process from
beginning to end.

Thus this book only provides guidelines for conducting research. The
framework on which it is based is illustrated in Fig. 1.1, but it must be
emphasized that this is a guide and not set in tablets of stone. Each

therapist must develop her own way of doing her research. As Evans (1978: 69) commented:

> The only way to learn to write is by writing, and the only way to learn research is by doing it oneself.

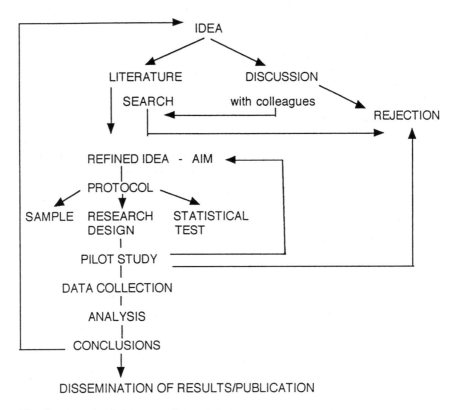

The framework of the research programme.

Preparation for research | 1

1.1 THE IDEA (THE OVERALL AIM OF RESEARCH)

A good question is one whose answer will matter.

Howie (1978)

Where do you begin? The flippant answer would be 'with an idea', an hypothesis, the 'what?' of the study. Where do you get the idea from? The simple answer to this question is either it comes to you or you must go and actively look for it. The first of these is obviously the easier option.

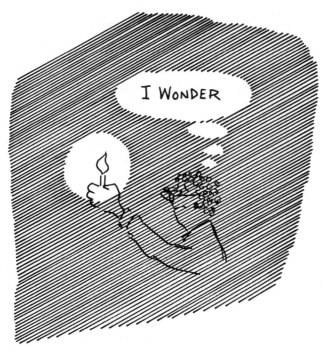

Figure 1.1 The idea.

Through personal observations, talking to colleagues and patients, or reading professional literature you notice a problem or a situation that intrigues you. This could cover anything: possible examples might be:

Why do patients with rheumatoid arthritis (RA) who are treated on one particular ward seem to do better than other patients with the same problems?

Would treatment A be just as successful delivered in a group setting as it is when it is used with individuals?

The second option, of actively looking for an idea, is more difficult, particularly so when a research topic has to be produced by a specific deadline. Unfortunately such deadlines have a habit of dulling rather than stimulating our thought patterns!

First you must decide on an area of interest. This is usually based on personal preference and resources. It would obviously be impractical to decide to look at recovery after amputation if you worked in a psychiatric setting. After selecting this area of interest – which can be as broad a category as 'neurology', 'orthopaedics', 'the elderly' – you must saturate yourself with information. You must talk to colleagues and patients, read, attend lectures and listen to the topical problems that are being discussed around you, such as:

- the effect on patients' treatment of ambulances being late

- the effect on social services of long hospital waiting lists.

Remember that you do not have to do something unique. You may well choose to develop research initiated by someone else. This can be done by changing the patient group, the staff group or even the type of treatment used. For example:

- it has been demonstrated that type B treatment is successful with patients with multiple sclerosis. Could it be used with the same success for patients with Parkinson's disease?

- patients respond to ultrasound when treated three times weekly. Would the result be the same if they were treated only twice weekly?

Remember that initial ideas will be more of a candle-flicker than a dazzling light.

A common problem many people have is the desire to make an idea more impressive or glamorous than it really is. Do not overestimate what you will be able to do. Keep your idea as simple as possible: try to clarify it and state it as clearly as possible. Many students who discuss their ideas with me often complain that it 'is too difficult to explain'. If it is too difficult to explain, it is too difficult to study.

A sound piece of advice: try to write down your idea in a sentence or as a question. If you cannot clarify the problem in this way, you will never clarify it. Putting something in writing often helps to narrow down the idea behind it into something more manageable. Consider the following as a facetious example: I have noted that many of my colleagues have spots. How can I narrow down my research idea and clarify exactly what I mean? The first step is to write down the idea and check each word.

Thus my research idea is: '*All therapists have acne.*'

'*All therapists*'
Q. Do I actually mean *all* therapists: OTs, physios, speech and language therapists?
A. No, I meant occupational therapists.
We can therefore revise our idea to '*All occupational therapists have acne.*'

Q. Do I mean *all* OTs?
A. No, I mean basic grade OTs working at my hospital.
Thus '*All basic grade occupational therapists at St John's Hospital have acne.*'

'*acne*'
Q. What do I mean by acne? Do I mean a clinical diagnosis of acne, or spots?
A. I mean spots.

By writing down the idea, modifying and revising it, the original idea can be narrowed to: 'All basic grade occupational therapists working at St John's Hospital have spots.' We can continue to break the idea down even further to make the aim more specific and the hypothesis more manageable. It is also important to consider the ideas behind what we are considering. That is, we must have some suggestions as to why the basic grade therapists have spots in the first place. It could be:

● Stress. Is this their first job after qualifying? Is there any difference in the number of spots in therapists who have been qualified for more than six months and those who are newly qualified? What evidence exists to suggest that stress produces spots?

● Chocolate. The therapists are continually receiving gifts of chocolate from grateful patients. Is there any differences between the number of spots in therapists who work on wards where less chocolate is received? Again, what evidence exists to suggest that eating chocolate produces spots?

● Environment. Do the therapists who work in the hospital have more spots than their counterparts who work in the community? Is there a relationship between developing spots and working in a hot, poorly ventilated environment?

Although this example is facetious, the principle behind the development of any research idea is fundamentally the same. All the words used and their meaning must be considered carefully before the hypothesis can be stated formally.

There is one further way in which you may get an idea for an investigation: your employer may give you a particular research field, with or without specifying an hypothesis. Most of the earlier advice about refining your question(s), working on simple ideas, writing down ideas and ensuring that your reserach proposal is manageable, applies just as much to studies prompted by your employer.

Hypothesis (note that the plural is 'hypotheses')

The Concise Oxford Dictionary defines hypothesis as:

> proposition made as basis for reasoning, without assumption of its truth; supposition made as a starting point for further investigation from known facts.

It is simply the term used in research for an idea. By tradition the hypothesis is always stated in terms of a relationship between two factors.

> There is a relationship between spots and the working environment.

The hypothesis and the null hypothesis are simply opposite sides of the same coin. Our example would then become:

> There is no relationship between spots and the working environment.

In a world where it is foolish to claim that anything can be proved beyond doubt, it is more realistic to be able to reject a negative relationship than it is to find sufficient evidence to support a positive one.

Cormack (1984: 56) rightly points out that some ideas are unanswerable because there is no right or wrong answer. To apply his point in a healthcare setting we might say it would be impossible to find out by research whether therapists *should* strike for better pay. The use of the word 'should' shows that the question is looking for a value judgement rather than a factual answer. However, asking this sort of unanswerable question can lead to spin-off ideas, for example:

> What are therapists' attitudes to striking?
> What are therapists' opinions on their level of pay?

Cormack believes the ideas that come from unresearchable topics can increase our understanding of the issues involved and help future decisions.

1.1.1 Sounding out the idea with colleagues

After clarifying the idea in your own mind, the next step i with your professional colleagues. Talk to anyone who will listen – tutors, work colleagues, those with and without research experience: the list is endless. Such discussion will help you to continue to modify your idea, make you aware of potential difficulties and perhaps add to the knowledge you already have. It is also valuable at this point to consult experts in your area of interest. They will have specific knowledge and essential information about the subject. They will also be in a better position to judge whether or not the idea is feasible to test.

It may be that having consulted all these individuals you realize that your study will not work. If this happens, do not get discouraged or defeated; your time has been well spent. It is much better to appreciate that an idea is too difficult to research or has already been exhaustively covered at this point, rather than several months into the research.

There are some words of caution, however, about sounding out your ideas. First, remember that some individuals will always be negative and pessimistic about research. You must decide whether to proceed on the basis of weighing up the information collected from a variety of people. Second, in the initial stages, care should be taken that a good research idea is not sounded out to others who might be tempted to use it themselves. Remember:

A clear question must be posed before the research is planned.

Huth (1982)

1.2 LITERATURE REVIEW

The literature review is part of the preparation process in planning a piece of research. Unfortunately many students misguidedly think the review is part of the method section of their project and consequently have serious problems as a result of leaving it until later in the study.

I must confess to being amused when I read papers where the author states that she has done a literature review. This is such an implicit part of the research process that it does not have to be said. It is assumed this has been done in the same way that recipes assume you crack the shells of eggs before using them. Do not expect to impress your readers or score extra Brownie points by stating this.

The literature review must reflect the author's knowledge of her field of interest; it involves searching for references and then sieving out the relevant information. The three sections involved in reviewing the literature for a study will be considered separately:

1.2.1 The literature search
1.2.2 Reviewing literature critically
1.2.3 Keeping records of references

1.2.1 The literature search

There are four main reasons for carrying out a literature search:

1. To show the extent of literature related to your field of interest but to ensure that there are no previous studies exactly like the one you are proposing. This avoids wasting valuable resources repeating a study that someone else has already carried out and it underlines the importance of your research.
2. To have up-to-date knowledge of relevant work in the field.
3. To identify factors you had not previously considered that could generate new questions.
4. To provide ideas on methods of investigation that could be used in your research.

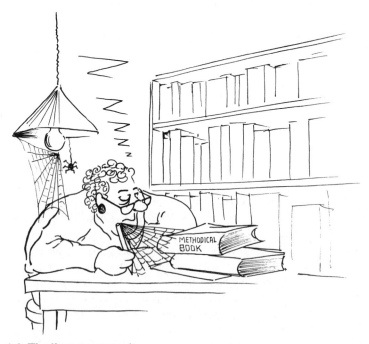

Figure 1.2 The literature search.

How do you find out what published literature is relevant to your study? A superficial search is important to give you the 'feel' of the area you are looking at and may even stimulate you to ask further questions or modify existing ideas. Such a search is done by obtaining references and information on your topic from:

- colleagues
- experts in the field
- references at the end of articles you have already found
- lists of further reading at the end of relevant book chapters and articles
- relevant journals, for example, if you are doing a study involving patients with Cerebral Vascular Accident (CVA) you could consult 'Stroke'. Similarly, if you are looking at a specific type of physiotherapy, you should scan through the physiotherapy journals
- dictionaries
- references and quotations given at meetings and lectures
- other dissertations.

However, although the superficial search is important initially, it is not satisfactory for a research project. For this you must carry out a more comprehensive search in order to identify all the relevant published literature. To do an in-depth search, you need access to a good medical library and, in the early stages, a helpful librarian. Do not rely on merely 'popping-in' to the library in the misguided hope that someone will be able to devote an hour to you. Ring up and make an appointment to see the librarian who deals with literature searches. Do not be tempted to explain your work over the telephone; you need to discuss your work in detail.

One final word of caution. Learn how to do the search yourself. The librarian who goes off to do it for you may be wonderful but is not helping you in the long run.

Sources of information

Journals
Journals are an essential source of information to the researcher. About 10 000 journals that are relevant to medicine are published throughout the world (Roberts, D., 1990). Indeed, it has been estimated that they account for 80% of the stock in a library (British Medical Association, 1987). However, because so many journals are published annually, tools are needed in order to find the information efficiently. These tools are known as indexes and abstracts. Quite simply, an indexing journal gives basic details of a reference while an abstracting journal provides a summary of the article.

The most widely used tools in medical circles are *Index Medicus* and *Excerpta Medica*. Although the paramedical literature is not particularly well covered by these tools (for example, several well-known physiotherapy and occupational therapy journals are not included) they are still, nevertheless, a valuable source of information to the research therapist.

Index Medicus

This is the most important indexing journal in medicine and is consequently stocked by virtually every medical library. It is produced in Washington by the National Library of Medicine and is published monthly. As *Index Medicus* draws on over 3000 medical and paramedical journals, it provides a comprehensive literature index. Articles are indexed according to subject and author.

A *Cumulated Index Medicus* is published annually. This lists all the articles that have been indexed in the previous 12 issues. Note that this does not only contain articles for the year indicated. As it may take several months for an article to be indexed, articles from the previous year will be included. For example, the 1992 *Cumulated Index Medicus* will contain some articles published in 1991.

A *List of Journals Indexed* is also published annually to give the full titles of the journals, which appear in an abbreviated form in the *Index*. It is vital to consult the abbreviations used for journals unless you are positive you know what they mean. Much time can be lost by looking for references that do not exist.

Conducting a search using *Index Medicus* The best way to learn how to do a search is with a librarian or a well-informed colleague. More detailed information on conducting a search can be found in Roberts, D. (1990).

Stages in carrying out a search

1. Find the *key words* in your idea. For example: 'An investigation of trigeminal neuralgia in multiple sclerosis'. The key words are: trigeminal neuralgia and multiple sclerosis.
2. Use the correct headings under which articles are indexed. These are called MeSH headings (Medical Subject Headings). If you do not use the appropriate headings, you will miss relevant information. Look up the MeSH headings for the key words: these may be different from what you expected. For example, if you look up 'Stroke' you will find: Stroke *see* Cerebrovascular disorders. Similarly, for 'Guillain-Barré syndrome' you will find: Guillain-Barré syndrome *see* Polyradiculoneuritis. These are the words you need to use in order to carry out your search.
3. Remember that some terms have been changed over the years and may have been listed differently in the past. *Index Medicus* will alert you to this. For example, if you are interested in publications on bulimia before 1987, you will be directed to look under the word 'Hyperphagia'.

Another example is spondylolysis: you need to look under Spondylo-listhesis prior to 1991.

4. Look up associated topics. MeSH will direct you to relevant areas with the words *see related*. For example, if you look up smoking you will find: Smoking *see related*: Tobacco use disorder. For psychological stress you will find: Stress, Psychological *see related* Crowding, Life change events.

5. Remember that as *Index Medicus* is an American publication, some of the spelling will be different. For example, for Colour blindness you will need to look up Color blindness; for Paediatrics you need Pediatrics.

Finally, remember to *set boundaries* before you conduct your search. For example, boundaries of:

- Time. How many years are you interested in? The last ten? The last 20?
- Language. Do you want to know about all articles or only those in the English language? Look at the reference to check which language it is written in.
- Others. This could include specifics such as male/female, human/animal, adult/child depending on the area of interest.

Excerpta Medica

This is an abstracting journal. So as well as providing information such as author, title and journal it provides a summary of the article in English. *Excerpta Medica* is published in Amsterdam and covers more than 4700 journals. Since the journal is so large the majority of libraries that stock it tend only to subscribe to a few sections. It is published in 51 sections, each of which covers a different topic. For example, *Section 19: Rehabilitation and physical medicine*; *Section 68: Arthritis and rheumatism*. The language to access information is virtually the same as for *Index Medicus*.

A word of warning: check that an article is in English before you send for it unless you are fluent in other languages. The abstract will always be in English but the rest of the paper may not be.

Here is a list (it should not be considered exhaustive) of other useful information sources:

Biological abstracts As the name suggests this encompasses the biological sciences. It is published fortnightly and has more than 9000 listings covering broad subject areas such as genetics and experimental medicine. It produces annual cumulations.

Current awareness *Current Contents*, for example, is a weekly publication of the contents pages of other journals. The most relevant from our point of view is probably *Clinical Medicine* which lists some 900 titles.

CATS (Current Awareness Topic Searches) are published on a wide range of subjects in 12 monthly issues. They are produced from the British Library Information Services from CATS' database. For example:

Physiotherapy Index: ISSN 0950–6659
Occupational Therapy Index: ISSN 0950–6675
Rehabilitation Index: ISSN 0955–0984
Complementary Medicine Index: ISSN 0950–6667
Palliative Care Index: ISSN 0961–4591

The chief advantage of CATS literature is that it is up-to-date.

Specialist indexing journals These are available in limited subject areas such as Carcinogenesis Abstracts. As they are specialized they tend to be very specific and comprehensive.

Psychological abstracts Abstracts from more than 1000 journals are included in this publication. It addresses all aspects of psychology and there are 16 major classifications with subheadings.

Review articles Indexing and Abstracting journals do not assess the quality of the papers they list. To find out more about quality you need to consult appropriate review articles. These are usually written by an expert and are a good starting point, providing a balanced and detailed overview of the subject.

It has been estimated that only 3% or 4% of all scientific literature consists of review papers (Jenkins, 1985: 51). With this small percentage of review material, the tool has limitations as a support for the newcomer to scientific publications.

Non-medical scientific publications *Science Citation Index*, for example, is published six times a year and it lists 3000 scientific journals. Unlike the other indexes, it is indexed by citation. This is essentially a reversal of the usual procedure: the reader looks up the earliest reference and sees papers that have subsequently cited it. The Index assumes that the greater the number of citations, the greater the importance of the work. This assumption is open to challenge and debate.

Use of computers The literature search may be conducted by hand or by computer ('online' and CD-ROM). Although the latter is quicker it is important that you do some of the searching manually in order to get a 'feel' of your research area. It will also enable you to become familiar with the work of major authors in the field. The majority of medical libraries now have facilities for researchers to do their own literature searches online. This is a great advantage. Delegating the task causes difficulties because 'to make a satisfactory search the librarian needs to know as much about the topic as the medical researcher' (Barber, Barraclough and Gray, 1972).

Online searching is said to be expensive because of charges for the telephone connections, expenses incurred in printing-out references and the costs of library staff. However, Elman (1975) in a study comparing the cost and searching time between online and manual searches, concluded that there was little difference between the two. One of the major advantages of using a computer is that it is flexible and quick and you can combine separate topics and access the information common to both (Roberts, D., 1990). This is known as cross-referencing. You can also check details of the cross-referenced materials by viewing these on screen before deciding which books or articles to pursue.

The Medical Literature Analysis and Retrieval System (MEDLARS) was first introduced in 1964. The first online database started in the 1970s and was called MEDLARS On Line (MEDLINE). MEDLINE is a database for:

Index Medicus
Index to Dental Index
International Nursing Index
Hospital Literature Index.

The points made above (under *Index Medicus*) about the use of MeSH headings are relevant to the MEDLINE system.

There is a range of other databases you may find useful. These include:

EMBASE (Excerpta Medica)
SCISEARCH (Science Citation)
PSYCIINFO (Psychological Abstracts)
CINAHL (Cumulative Index of Nursing and Allied Health Literature).

Most medical libraries in teaching hospitals now have terminals where such databases can be accessed. This means that library users have 'more comprehensive, effective and relevant information services and teaching programmes' than in the past (Pentelow, 1989).

Books
Library book holdings are listed in catalogues. These range from simple card-filing systems to microfiche and Automated librarian online public access terminals (OPACS). Books can be listed under their subject, title, author or in a dictionary catalogue. In the latter system, subjects and names are listed in alphabetical order. Information can be found both by looking up the subject area or, if you know that someone is famous in a particular field, by looking up an author. All books are given a shelfmark so that you can find them efficiently.

Many libraries classify books under the Dewey Decimal Classification System. All books are divided into ten main classes according to topic, ranging from 000 to 999. All medical books are listed from 610–619 and each of these classes is subdivided again. Books with the same classmark are arranged in an alphabetical listing. For example:

600–699	Applied science
610–619	Medical
616	Diseases
616.8	Brain diseases
616.836	Cerebral palsy

Numbers that appear after a decimal point allow greater specificity. There are problems in this system in classifying some literature, for example government White Papers, so it is important to see how your library lists items you are unable to find.

Dissertations

This tends to be an overlooked area for literature searches. Valuable information can be obtained by consulting dissertations and they can direct you to other important references.

Dissertation Abstracts International This provides details and abstracts of theses/dissertations accepted in American and European universities. It is the most comprehensive list available.

Most countries have their own publication on dissertations, for example, *Great Britain and Ireland*:

Index of Theses Accepted for Higher Degrees by the Universities of Great Britain and Ireland (published by Aslib). Information from: Expert Information, Woodside, Hinksey Hill, Oxford OX1 5AU
USA
Comprehensive Dissertation Index. Information from: UMI – Dissertation Abstracts Online, 300 N. Zeeb Road, Annarbor, Michigan, MI 48106 U.S.

Inter-library loans

Libraries are unable to stock all the articles and books their readers want. Even if a library does keep a journal in which you are interested, you may find that a particular issue is missing. So it is an important role of the library to obtain literature it does not hold. Some libraries operate in geographical networks and have information about journals held in and readily accessible from neighbouring libraries. This is particularly useful where journals are not used regularly in all the libraries of a network.

The main source for loans is the British Library Document Supply

Centre in Boston Spa. This centre deals with other libraries (not individual readers) and has around 12 000 requests daily (*British Medical Association*, 1987). Although the service is efficient it is not cheap. It is wise to keep costs down by careful choice, based on looking at abstracts before asking for particular journal articles. Most libraries have special forms for requesting inter-library loans. Theses and dissertations from other universities can also be requested in this way.

Photocopying

The Copyright Act 1988 has strict rules about what and how much you can copy and for what purpose. It restricts the number of copies that can be made for research or private study to one article per issue of a periodical. When library users ask someone else (usually the librarian) to do their photocopying, they must sign a declaration to this effect. Libraries normally have their own forms for this purpose. It is also accepted practice that not more than one-tenth of a monograph or book may be copied.

Interestingly, it was not until I was researching this book that I realized that the law does not distinguish between the methods of copying used. It is still infringing copyright to copy a paper by hand without signing a copyright declaration (British Medical Association, 1987: 92).

Reprints

In some cases, reprints of published articles can be obtained by writing directly to the author. This usually occurs when researchers are unable to get photocopies of articles through the library service. However, it is becoming increasingly difficult to obtain reprints in this way because postage costs and the reduced availability of complimentary reprints to authors have made them less inclined to respond to such requests.

Serendipity

The Oxford Dictionary defines serendipity as 'the faculty of making happy and unexpected discoveries by accident'. You will never cease to be amazed at the number of times you will find exactly the information you want just by chance.

1.2.2 Reading literature critically

It is wise to debate and challenge the methods and findings of any article, however persuasive it is on first sight. Even if something is factually correct, there may be another equally acceptable viewpoint or interpretation. It is also important to make the point that rubbish does get into print.

Many people seem to find this a difficult concept to grasp as they believe that anything which appears in print must be true.

Reading an article critically is a skill, not one that comes naturally to most people but one that must be learned and practised. Journal clubs provide an excellent way of doing this by pooling ideas and comments on articles in an informal and non-threatening setting. Even if you feel there is nobody on your ward or in your department who would be able to lead such a group, do not be dissuaded. Enthusiasm is the most essential ingredient. The opinions of everyone are valuable and you will learn to view articles from different perspectives. As the group progresses and people become more confident of sharing their opinions, you may ask for input from someone you know is involved in research.

It is very useful (I would say essential) to have pen and paper at hand when you are reading an article. If it is not your own copy you must photocopy it before writing on the text in any way. As a personal preference I find highlighting pens of great help. Scan through the article. Underline the important points the author raises and highlight anything that interests you.

Parahoo and Reid (1988) comment that 'critical reading of research is an appraisal of its strengths and limitations'. It is all too easy to criticize someone else's work without attempting to look at the good points. If you fall into the trap of always looking at the negative side of papers you will become your own worst enemy. You will always be dissuaded from research because you only see the problems. You can say something good about every paper: even if you conclude that an article is appalling it has at least provided you with a useful teaching tool.

What do you look at when you read an article or piece of research? It is best to work methodically through the paper rather than trying to absorb everything at once.

Title

This should not affect your overall opinion of the article although it is nevertheless frustrating when the title does not reflect the content of the paper. Do not be discouraged by a poor title.

Introduction

This section should 'set the scene' for the article. The author should include a LITERATURE REVIEW to set the study in the context of previous work done in the area. When you are reviewing the introduction, consider the following:

- Does the author attempt to analyse and comment constructively on previous work or does she merely outline and use quotations from these studies?

- How recent are the studies that have been cited? That is, how up to date is the review?

- How relevant are these cited studies?

- Does the author use primary sources or is she content to give references cited by others? Does she note facts or opinions?

- Do you understand the background to the study and the need for the present investigation?

- Do you understand what the overall aim of the study is?

Finally, remember that although a poorly presented introduction reflects badly on the paper, it does not necessarily mean that the actual study is poor.

Methodology

This is one of the most important sections to read critically. If there are problems in the methodology, the whole study could be flawed. Although this section will be examined in greater detail in Chapters 2 and 3, the most important points to note are:

- Was the sample representative of the group being studied?

- Was the sample size adequate to prove or disprove an hypothesis?

- Were the outcome measures RELIABLE and VALID?

- Was the most appropriate method of investigation employed? For example, if you wanted to evaluate a treatment technique on range of movement, would sending a postal questionnaire to the patient be the best method of collecting data?

- If the most obvious method was not employed, were satisfactory reasons given for the method used?

- Could you repeat the study?

If any of these factors arouse uneasiness, the rest of the article should be read carefully in the context of your misgivings.

Results

This section should be factual with no opinions expressed by the author. Consider:

- Do any results appear to be missing?

- Is the statistical test applied (if any) appropriate? See section 5.4.

- Has the statistical test been used correctly? See section 5.4.

- Are the results presented in percentages and supported by the NUMBER of observations? Remember that 50% could be two subjects out of four.

- Is there any obvious bias?

- Is the hypothesis accepted or rejected?

Discussion

This part of the article should link in closely with the introduction. The author should attempt to place the findings of her study in the context of previous literature. Explanations should be suggested for the results obtained with particular reference to any difficulties encountered. It is valuable when authors offer a critique of their own methodology. Within the discussion, the author may present deductions which must be firmly supported by EVIDENCE, as well as opinions and speculations related to the findings.

Conclusions

Are the conclusions justified by the work presented in the results section? Remarkably this is an area where many research papers lose credibility: authors accept their original hypothesis despite evidence they present to the contrary. Often it is only possible 'to suggest' that the hypothesis can be supported or not or to say that a trend is identified. It is reasonable to be sceptical of an author who believes that her study 'proves' something.

Recommendations

It is important to check that these link in with what the results actually say. Even if the author does adhere to her findings, is it reasonable to make a major recommendation on the basis of the study?

An excellent paper by Fowkes and Fulton (1991) gives detailed guidelines and a checklist for critically appraising published research.

1.2.3 Keeping records of references

It is vital to keep accurate details about every article, journal and book you read in connection with your research. These details must include the author's surname and initials, the year of publication, the title of the book or article, city of publication and publisher or name of journal, volume and issue (see listed items below). Although recording seems tedious in the early stages, it soon becomes a habit which is easy to carry on. Time invested in this way saves the frustration later of searching for a valuable reference you have mislaid or initially did not think was of great importance.

Many researchers advocate the use of small record cards that can be stored in boxes. These cards can be arranged in alphabetical order (according to the author's surname) and are easily accessible and transportable. Alternatively, a record may be kept on computer, using a database that is easy to access. If a computerized reference list is created, it is essential to keep back-up copies on disks and to up-date them regularly. In setting up a reference database, it is wise to use keywords for subsequent cross-referencing (see Chapter 5).

The most important information to record is:

on books:

- author(s) surname and initials
- year of publication
- title of book and relevant chapter(s)
- place/city of publication
- name of publisher
- number of first and last pages.

on articles:

- author(s) surname and initials
- year of publication
- title of article
- title of journal
- volume
- issue
- number of first and last pages.

Although it may seem to save time initially, it is best to avoid using abbreviations when recording this information, unless you are using accepted journal abbreviations such as those used in *Index Medicus*. From personal experience I can assure you that it is just as frustrating to have a reference that you cannot make sense of as it is to have no reference at all.

Other information which may be recorded is:

- Whether you have a copy of the article/the source of reference. This is usually indicated by a tick or the name of a person/location where the book or reference can be found.

- Personal comments. For example, notes on how relevant the article is to your study, your opinion on the quality of the article ('poor', 'good', 'valuable') or any points you feel you would like to jot down. If you find that an article or book is completely irrelevant to your study, do not discard the reference. Note down all the details and your comments exactly as before. This will prevent you from thinking you have missed an important paper later in the study and wasting resources in tracing it again.

● Quotations. It is often useful to copy quotations EXACTLY from articles or to record important results on the back of record cards.

Wherever possible it is advisable to keep a copy of the articles you use (see page 13 on Photocopying). NEVER throw anything out: you may not appreciate its worth until much later. Original articles and photocopies should be stored in files in alphabetical order, preferably according to the author's name. If you store details according to subject you may have great problems if you are studying a very narrow field.

Finally, remember that PLAGIARISM (that is, stealing the writing and ideas of others and presenting them as your own) is a serious offence. It is important to reference the work of others accurately and credit their ideas where appropriate.

1.3   ETHICAL CONSIDERATIONS

Definition of ethics: Seaman (1987: 30) has defined ethics as 'the study and evaluation of human conduct'. *The Oxford Dictionary* states that it is both the 'science of morals' and the 'rules of conduct'. In practice, ethical principles are essentially a combination of law and professional convention. These principles are applied within healthcare and within the studies that support the development and improvement of that care. Decisions on contentious issues are taken by ethical committees whose remit is to protect people while enabling appropriate research.

> As a result of medical progress, our technical decisions may become easier but moral problems, on the contrary, will be increasingly significant.
>
> Hamburger (1968: 136)

In 1947 the World Medical Association produced ethical guidelines known as the *Declaration of Geneva*, after widespread concern was voiced about medical research undertaken by the Nazis during the Second World War. This is an international code of ethics which applies in both war and peace. In 1964 the World Medical Association published the *Declaration of Helsinki*. This was revised in 1975 and became known as *Helsinki II*. This formal code was written specifically for the guidance of doctors involved in human experimentation. The majority of medical and paramedical bodies in Europe and America have subsequently produced their own guidelines and professional codes of ethics, based on these declarations.

A useful rule of thumb for the researcher who is not sure whether a piece of proposed research is ethical is to ask the question 'How would I feel if I were the person involved in this study?' Remember that it is not enough to look at the situation from your own perspective. You must consider it from the cultural, racial, social and religious background of the potential subject. If you have any reservations in answering this question you need to look again at the style and content of the proposed research.

Remember also to assess the POTENTIAL risks involved. Currier (1984) underlines that 'research often involves uncertainties which may in turn involve risks'. Similarly, remember that potential risks are not just the physical implications of research, such as discomfort or pain. Psychological effects, such as embarrassment or emotional upset, must also be considered.

1.3.1 The ethical committee

ALL research that involves, or is likely to involve, patients or staff should be submitted for ethical approval. Ethical committees are usually multi-disciplinary and consist of doctors, nurses, administrators and lay people. The role of the committee is to act as a watchdog to ensure that the best interests of individuals are represented and that patients and staff are not subjected to unnecessary risks. Some committees are both research and ethical committees. They are therefore responsible for monitoring the standard of the proposed research in addition to making sure that there are no problems of an ethical nature.

Proposals are usually submitted to the secretary or chairperson of the committee at least one month before the date of the next meeting. In some instances, particularly where ethical considerations are minor, there is provision for the chairperson to approve projects without consulting the rest of the committee. The documentation pertaining to ethical approval should be kept safely for future reference. Ethical and research proposals are dealt with in detail in section 1.5 below.

1.3.2 Specific considerations

There are some specific considerations which are accepted practice in research unless it has been agreed otherwise at a local level.

1. Subjects have the right to remain anonymous. The researcher must protect the identity of subjects throughout the study and in any publication of the final work. This is often achieved by allocating

subjects a number and keeping the code to the names separately and securely.

2. The information collected is confidential. Any information collected on subjects must be kept safely and not disclosed to anyone outside the study. Subjects must also be informed if information is going to be placed in a computer. Provision for the rights of subjects is contained in the Data Protection Act (1984). Researchers have a legal obligation to observe the requirements of this Act.
3. Individuals may be approached to participate in a study but it is their right to refuse. They must be free from any form of coercion.
4. Subjects are free at any stage in the project (even if this would prove disastrous to the research) to withdraw without prejudice.
5. All the information collected must relate to the study.
6. The research must be conducted by researchers who are recognized as competent.
7. The research must be justifiable for scientific value. However, even if this criterion is met, the potential benefits should not be outweighed by the potential risks.
8. The consent of the doctor who has overall responsibility for the patient is required.
9. If treatment is known to be effective it is unethical to withhold it from patients. However, if the effect of a type of treatment is unknown or unclear, it has been argued that it is unethical NOT to evaluate it. Makrides and Richman (1981) note the difficulties that many therapists have in accepting 'control' or 'no treatment' groups in studies but comment 'If the treatment is *considered* to be beneficial – *without the clinician knowing for sure* – continued use of the treatment without proper assessment of its value is considered unethical' (my italics).

   On the other hand, it is generally accepted that patients derive some benefit by virtue of the fact that they are receiving some treatment: thus there is an *attentional* effect. It may therefore be argued that to withhold all treatment input is depriving the patient of some aspect of care. Both these ideas have important implications for the investigation of a variety of paramedical treatments which have been used for many years and which now need to be researched.
10. Bad research is unethical: it misleads others throughout the world and may prevent someone else carrying out a thorough investigation of the topic.

1.3.3 Informed consent

Subjects can only be involved in a research project if they have given their consent. Moreover, it is the responsibility of the researcher to ensure that the person is able to take this decision with all the information available.

Potential subjects must be made aware that their participation is voluntary and that they may withdraw at any time. They must be told about the time and nature of any treatments and of any possible risks. They should also be given the opportunity to ask questions. Never assume that an individual is willing to participate in a study.

Withholding consent

In some instances a full explanation of a research project might alter the behaviour or responses of the subjects being studied. Consequently the results would be affected. The Royal College of Physicians (1990) accepts that 'there are some circumstances in which it is justifiable to initiate research without the consent of the patient' but notes: 'Such circumstances do not affect the duty of the investigator to obtain the prior approval of the Research Ethics Committee in the usual way.'

Documentation

In the past, subject permission was given orally. The trend today, with greater emphasis on litigation, is to obtain written consent. In such instances patients and staff are asked to sign a consent form which may also be signed by the researcher. Such forms should be stored and kept safely.

Additional measures that may be taken in seeking oral and written consent are issuing patient-information sheets about the research; allowing patients time for reflection; obtaining witnessed consent and inviting a

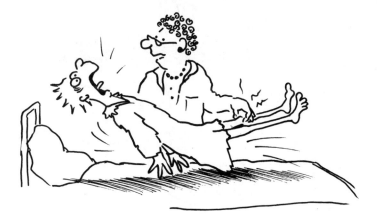

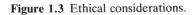

You did say you would help didn't you!

Figure 1.3 Ethical considerations.

third party to act as an advisor to the patient (Royal College of Physicians, 1990).

Ethics and ethical considerations present complex issues in their own right. There is no accepted framework that is agreed by all researchers but there are some areas where the majority agree. Outside these areas the researcher must stay within her professional code of conduct and be able to account for and justify her actions.

1.4   FINANCIAL CONSIDERATIONS

There are many practical considerations to be taken into account when planning a research project. It will come as little surprise to most therapists in the present economic climate to learn that most of these concern money.

1.4.1   Costing the project

Why do you need to cost a research project? First, if you are applying for funds you will need to know how much money you need to complete the project. You must ensure that you have not underestimated the amount involved. Second, it must be established that the project is financially viable. It would be a waste of money, for example, to research a treatment that is rarely used.

It is necessary to consider both CAPITAL COSTS (one-off expenses) and

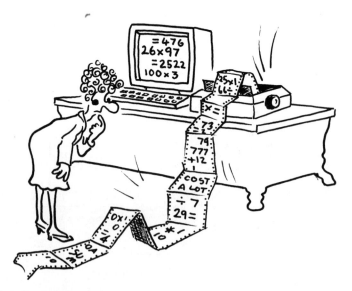

Figure 1.4 Costing the project.

RECURRENT COSTS. Since every research project is different, it is impossible to outline every specific consideration. However, the following is a useful checklist:

- salaries: include pension and health-insurance contributions
- secretarial support
- travel: include your costs, those of subjects and those of the independent assessor. Do not forget the cost to the ambulance service, if applicable
- new equipment
- new materials
- computer disks and the use of computer facilities
- stationery
- photocopying
- postage
- telephone and fax
- the cost of library service: obtaining references, online searches
- the cost of registration, if your research is to be used for a higher degree.

When costing recurrent expenses it is important to remember the length of time that will be involved. Remember to consider increases in salaries and travel as a result of pay awards and inflation. If you are concerned about the cost analysis that you are undertaking, you can get advice and assistance from the hospital finance department.

Even if you do not feel that the research will cost anything, run through this checklist. Your time is money, so if you are going to devote three hours a week to the research, remember that that is three hours' salary. Do not underestimate the amount of TIME you will need to spend on the project. In addition to the actual time spent conducting the investigation, you must allow for other aspects of the study. For example:

- completing application forms (for the finance or the ethical committee)
- attending interviews, both formal (such as with the ethical committee) and informal (meeting with a consultant to ask for assistance)
- checking ward admissions
- visiting the library
- travelling from place to place
- analysing and writing up your results.

Also remember the amount of time potentially involved in receiving permission to do the study, in obtaining money and actually setting up the investigation.

1.4.2 Applying for grants and finance

Ask for what you need to do the job at hand. Use common sense.

Merritt (1963)

Unless you find yourself in the position of being appointed to a research post, you will be faced with the prospect of applying for funding. This can be for varying amounts that may include:

- covering the fees for a further education course
- paying your salary while you undertake a research project
- covering the expenses of an entire research project
- paying for additional or new equipment
- a contribution towards expense costs.

WHO do you apply to for finance?

Health authority

If you wish to undertake your project at work, even if you do not need additional funding, you must seek permission and approval from your line manager. Remember that your time is expensive.

If you do require funding from your health authority, investigate any research funds they may have such as regional or local research grants. Check hospital noticeboards and contact health authority headquarters. Most authorities have a research policy and employ an individual who is responsible for helping prospective researchers.

Companies

If you wish to evaluate a particular piece of equipment, it may be worth while contacting the company that produces it. It may be difficult to have an expensive item of equipment at your disposal if other therapists need it. Thus it would make good sense to try to 'borrow' one for your research.

In the medical field the drug companies provide large sums of money for research. Although their profit margins are not in the same league, the majority of companies who rely on therapists to buy their equipment donate relatively little to research. However, that should not deter you from asking them for help, particularly when it is to evaluate their products.

Specific charities

If you are interested in researching the effects of a particular condition, you may be able to apply for help to the charity most involved. Examples include The Stroke Association, The Rheumatism and Arthritis Council, Asthma Research, British Heart Foundation and Action for the Crippled Child. Some charities advertise annual bursaries.

Generic funding

There are several avenues to investigate regarding general funding for research. Examples include the Department of Health and Social Security,

The Kings' Fund, The Medical Research Council, Science Research Council, Social Science Research Council. Some of these advertise research training awards.

Assistance from professional bodies
It is good to develop the habit of scanning the professional journals. Most therapy and nursing bodies offer funds to contribute towards research costs. All the awards are different and the conditions of each must be read carefully, but they usually offer a lump sum that can be used for equipment, research expenses or registration for a qualification.

University assistance
As each university is different the situation will vary enormously from region to region. However, it is worth while pursuing local bursaries that might be available, for example, for postgraduate research projects. Particular departments may also be able to help with finance for research in particular fields.

Interest-free loans

Anyone who might give you money
A copy of the *Charities Digest* will be found in any good library. This is a valuable book to consult if you are looking for funding. It is usually held as a reference book, so go to the library with lots of paper, an extra pen and time to spare. There is no easy way to consult this book but the best idea is to scan through it. You will be surprised at the number of charities that outline conditions that may be relevant to you. You must read this book for yourself and not rely on others. You will find, for example, that you are eligible to apply for finance on the basis of the occupations of other family members – which obviously may not apply to other colleagues. Never dismiss anything before examining it carefully.

Other useful publications include the *Research Funds Guide*, *Directory of Grant-Making Trusts*, *Grants Register* and the *Handbook of the Association of Medical Research Charities*. There may also be some merit in checking medical research centres and the world directory of organizations and programmes.

Finally, remember to ask other colleagues in research how they obtained their funding.

How do you apply for funds?

The British Medical Association commented in 1971 that 'There is no doubt that a worthwhile research project sometimes fails to obtain financial support because of the manner in which the application for it is presented.' This is just as true today. Applications for finance need to be treated with the same reverence as those for jobs. Merritt (1963) coined the phrase 'grantsmanship' to describe the art of lucid presentation she outlines in her excellent paper.

Allen (1960) described the characteristic shortcomings of rejected applications for funds. His review concluded that the majority of applications were rejected because of problems in describing the actual aim of the proposed study and the approach to be taken. Applying for funding is highly competitive, so the quality of the whole proposal is important. Individuals who judge the application are responsible for distributing the money at their disposal wisely to individuals with promising studies. They are usually experts in their field and you should never underestimate their knowledge.

Guidelines on applying for funds to charities, firms and companies

Where no application form is available (or none is supplied)

- Send a letter written in legible handwriting or typed (but signed personally), addressed whenever possible to a named individual. You should outline:
  WHY you are writing (what are you researching?)
  HOW MUCH money you need
  The VALUE of researching this area (the value to them).

- Include an up-to-date curriculum vitae. This demonstrates your ability to do the research and makes you a distinctive individual. For information on writing a good curriculum vitae I recommend O'Brien (1990) or Jones (1990).

- Where possible, send a stamped addressed envelope (sae). This should guarantee a reply and, if your request is unsuccessful, many agencies will return your CV to be used again.

Where an application form is supplied
Some larger organizations and charities will provide an application form to be completed. Photocopy it immediately so that you can practise the layout of your answers. Remember:

- Complete the form as requested (typed, black ink)

- Answer all questions. If a question is not relevant write N/A (not applicable). Do not just leave it blank.

- Do not merely put 'see attached CV' in response to questions about your career. Answer questions in the spaces provided and attach an appendix if you need to write more.

- Respond using the headings given. When outlining your proposal, amend any wording you have used before. For example, do not use the heading 'method' if the heading given is 'plan of investigation'.

- Many charities now ask for application forms to be photocopied. If this is requested, do not forget to include the correct number.

- It is polite to include a covering letter or compliment slip with your completed application form.

Some further tips

- Submit your application form as early as possible.

- Tailor your application to the agency from whom you are requesting assistance.

- Prove that you have the necessary qualities/facilities/support to conduct the project.

- Ask an experienced colleague to read and comment on your application.

- Do not despair or be deterred if your request is rejected. This happens to all researchers. If you feel there is a problem in the proposal, it may be useful to seek feedback. However, it could simply be that the agency is already funding a project similar to yours.

1.5   WRITING A PROTOCOL

The protocol, which may also be called the proposal, has been defined by Currier (1984) as 'a document that outlines a planned project or investigation'. Thus it is simply a written plan of the research project. Such a plan is necessary:

- to have a reference document that sets limits. This helps you as the researcher to adhere to your original plan. It is easy to get sidetracked from the original investigation, particularly if your research is likely to take you a long time.

- in order to have an overview of the entire project. Inaccuracies or details that need attention often come to light during the writing of the proposal.

- to gain an entrée where the researcher is relatively unknown or where a new line of research is proposed.

- to submit to an ethical committee.

- to submit for funding or sponsorship.

As already mentioned, some committees and organizations have their own forms or provide specific criteria for the proposal. However, where this is not provided the outline below can be used as a guide of what must be included.

1.5.1 Content of the protocol

The protocol should:

- follow a logical sequence
- give a broad outline of the proposed study
- include as much detail as necessary to answer obvious queries
- avoid the use of jargon or specialized technical words
- not exceed six sides of A4. Long protocols are not read in detail.

It must include:

1. A title that pinpoints the subject being researched. Avoid both a long, detailed title and a short ambiguous one. Remember your aim is to be informative. You are not trying to find the wittiest, flashiest title.
2. A brief outline of present knowledge in the field. The proposal should reflect the researcher's appreciation of other work carried out in the area.
3. The aim of the proposed study. If it is not obvious why the research is needed from the review of literature, this must be explained and justified.
4. The method of study. This should include information on the numbers of subjects needed, the selection of these subjects, the data to be collected, the method of collecting data and the method of analysis.
5. Ethical considerations, particularly in protocols to be submitted to ethical committees. Even the most obvious points should be stated, for example that subjects are free to withdraw from the study at any time. Any potential risks must be identified and justified.
6. The value or effect of the study should be considered. You should outline the effects of a study which may change current practice or have major professional implications.
7. Costs (if applicable). Details must be included on both capital and recurrent costs (see 1.4.1).
8. References. These are not essential although their inclusion may strengthen the points you raise.

Do not send the same protocol to every organization. It is important that you emphasize the significant points that are relevant to each individual organization. For example, a proposal to an ethical committee should emphasize ethical considerations, whereas a proposal for money should seek to provide comprehensive financial details of the study. Similarly it is important to use the headings provided by the organization. For example, if the heading 'Plan of investigation' is given, do not use your own heading of 'Method' or 'Methodology'. In practice, with increased access to word processors, such alterations do not take a great deal of time as often only minor changes are needed. The extra work is always worth while.

2	# The research process

2.1 INTRODUCTION

Continuing the issue of planning a study, this chapter addresses the scope of research methodology and explores the elements that need to be considered before important decisions can be made. In the sections below, you will find details of:

- the DESIGN of an investigation. Five options are outlined

- the SELECTION OF SUBJECTS, with a detailed introduction of sampling routines and criteria for inclusion and exclusion

- the NUMBERS of subjects to be recruited, with emphasis on the interactions between the design of a study and the size of a sample population.

2.2 DESIGN OF THE STUDY

> The word design implies the organisation of elements into a masterful work of art.
>
> LoBiondo-Wood and Haber (1990: 128)

> Bad experimental designs create problems that cannot be corrected by any statistical procedure, however sophisticated.
>
> Shott (1990)

Burns and Grove (1987: 228) rightly discuss the problem that many researchers have with regard to the use of the word 'design'. They point out that some individuals use it to refer to the whole strategy for their studies. In this book the term is used in the way they explain it as 'clearly defined structural frameworks within which the study is implemented'.

Beginning a study without a design is like going shopping without a list:

frustrating, purposeless and with a strong risk of overlooking something. A design provides the foundation for the entire study, so the choice of design is critical. You must select the design that is most appropriate to your study and that others will recognize and accept as suitable. Remember that there may be a number of designs that you could use. It is your responsibility to choose the best one.

Which is the best? Quite simply, the best design is the one that allows you to collect the information you need in order to answer your original research. Whenever feasible it is preferable to work with designs that have been used successfully before. In many instances, you will come across suitable designs as you sift through the literature in your field of interest.

Before planning an investigation, you should consider the options of style, time reference and subject choice that are available in a range of research designs. You must decide whether to choose:

- descriptive or interventive studies
- experimental or correlational designs
- retrospective or prospective studies
- cross-sectional or longitudinal designs
- single or group studies.

2.2.1 Descriptive or interventive studies

You must decide whether you wish to describe a situation as it occurs or whether you wish to intervene. Let us consider these choices separately.

Descriptive studies

Description is an essential stage in establishing a professional knowledge base.

Partridge and Barnitt (1986)

The overall aim of a descriptive study is to describe a situation or practice in order to gain additional information. By using this design, information is collected on what occurs naturally in the 'real life' situation. Descriptive studies often provide a valuable baseline for further investigations because they enable us to define what actually happens. For example, before conducting a research project on the effectiveness of Bobath treatment, you may need to carry out a descriptive study in order to explain the meaning of the term 'Bobath therapy'.

Descriptive studies are also important for identifying problems in practice, for justifying current practice and for developing theory (Waltz and Bausall, 1981, in Burns and Grove, 1987). For example, you may describe a service to illustrate how it succeeds or describe a service to identify its shortcomings.

Interventive studies

Some researchers argue that to intervene in any situation brings about change and therefore you are not studying the real situation. However, much research explores situations that involve the need to intervene. In these cases, the researcher plans and records the necessary interventions, making these as realistic and clinically relevant as possible. A particular style of study known as 'action research' recognizes and formalizes this focus. Within nursing in particular, studies have been designed to feed back the details of care that seemed to be effective in the first phase of a project into a formal treatment regime for the next phase of observation.

2.2.2. Experimental or correlational designs

Experimental designs

> The experimental design is intended to ensure that an experiment affords a valid, efficient and unambiguous test of the hypothesis set up and that extraneous variables are controlled.
>
> Miller and Wilson (1983)

Experimental designs are not commonly used in social sciences or in treatment settings, as it is often difficult to translate the findings into realistic implications for practice. The important factor about this is that as many variables as possible are controlled so that the effect of one variable on another can be investigated. The researcher attempts to manipulate a variable (the INDEPENDENT VARIABLE) in order to assess the effect on another variable (the DEPENDENT VARIABLE, i.e. its performance is dependent on the factor being manipulated).

For example, suppose a therapist wished to evaluate whether an education programme for patients having a total hip replacement (THR) could reduce the number of post-operative dislocations. In this situation, the education programme (the treatment) would be the independent variable and the number of dislocations recorded would be the dependent variable.

The whole environment must be carefully controlled in such a study so that no other factors are allowed to interfere. It may therefore be concluded that any result is due to the manipulated factor. In an experimental design, the researcher attempts to examine relationships by looking at the DIFFERENCES between results. The researcher is interested in CAUSE and EFFECT, but may not be able to record more than the coexistence of the independent variable and a range of observed events. To meet some of the special needs for the evaluation of treatments and techniques, adaptations of experimental design known as randomized controlled trials (RCT) have been developed. These and the older more traditional experimental approach, known simply as clinical trials, are discussed further in Chapter 3.

Correlational designs

If an experimental design looks at differences, correlational designs concentrate on RELATIONSHIPS. In contrast to the manipulated conditions of an experimental study, those of a correlational study are not varied by the plans of the researcher. In other words, there are no independent or dependent variables. The researcher studies the situation in search of associations and links. Once these are observed and recorded, the resulting patterns of relationships can be analysed and clarified. Although some relationships may be suggested by looking at the results, it is unwise to speculate about correlations without using suitable statistical tests and their interpretations (see Chapter 5).

2.2.3 Retrospective or prospective studies

Retrospective studies

A retrospective study is one in which 'the investigator looks back from apparent effects to preceding causes' (Cooke, 1980). In this type of study, the researcher assembles and analyses PAST information. For example, she consults the past medical records of a group of patients with the same diagnosis. Retrospective studies can provide valuable information about the achievements of a particular service. For example, Kaye (1991) conducted an audit of physiotherapy records at a London hospital using 20 records selected at random from recent discharges. The records were used to explore problems, goals and outcomes for these discharged people.

Information can be collected relatively quickly in this type of study, but there is a danger that records may be inaccurate or incomplete. Some information may be based on memories reported by people: such memories may be distorted and cannot be checked.

Prospective studies

Prospective studies identify 'putative causes at one time point' (Cooke, 1989) and monitor people to see who is affected by the identified factors and who is not. We can find an example of a prospective study in the work of N.A. Roberts (1990) who followed up elderly patients after their discharge from the accident and emergency department of a large hospital.

Although more conclusive results can be obtained in a prospective investigation than in a retrospective study, there are fewer potential sources of bias and data collection costs both time and money.

2.2.4   Cross-sectional or longitudinal designs

Cross-sectional designs

The researcher studies subjects in the same time period but at different stages or levels of involvement. These studies attempt to measure cause and effect while focusing on things that are happening simultaneously. Such studies are likely to be used most widely. Results are obtained quickly but there may be problems in interpreting them or in generalizing the research findings to a wider population than the one representative in a particular study.

Kirkwood (1988: 155) comments that 'cross-sectional studies are relatively quick, cheap and easy to carry out, and straightforward to analyse'. Such a study could involve asking patients about their experience in hospital or asking qualified staff about their professional education or training.

Longitudinal designs

Longitudinal studies attempt to measure cause and effect occurring at different points of time. Such studies can provide evidence but not explanations of what happens. They cannot be used to infer anything beyond the results and effects that are actually recorded.

The major difficulty with longitudinal studies lies in the problems of following up subjects over long periods of time. Many factors can change and affect the situation. In epidemiology, samples from time-dimensional studies are known as COHORTS. The researcher focuses on the same specific population but this may alter over time: some subjects may be lost and others gained. The nature and numbers of a cohort may therefore change.

To illustrate the difference between cross-sectional and longitudinal studies, we consider two projects to investigate the effect of a treatment on people with multiple sclerosis (MS). One project, planned for a two-week period in the spring of 1995, looks at patients receiving treatment at that time, those who have just completed their treatment and a further group who finished their treatment programme six months ago (cross-sectional study). The other project has selected a cohort of people with MS and will follow them over a two-year period, observing them repeatedly at six-week intervals (longitudinal study).

2.2.5 Single or group studies

There have been many debates between researchers about whether it is 'better' research to use single or group designs. Some people seem to suggest that you must make a choice between the two: either you always use a group or you always have a single subject design. Frankly, this is nonsense: the two are complementary and neither is intrinsically better than the other. A single subject study can be the basis for a group design. Similarly, if a group design demonstrates that a treatment is effective, a single subject study can be used to investigate the implications for an individual.

Single studies

Sunderland (1990) underlines the importance of distinguishing between a CASE STUDY and a SINGLE CASE EXPERIMENT. He defines the first of these not as an experiment at all, but as 'retrospective reports of observations made on interesting individual patients'. Case studies may thus be used to provide clues for future clinical evaluations and their detailed observations can be fed into a pool of empirical evidence.

Single case designs involve the study of a unit (an individual, a family) and the effect of a large number of variables. As long as such studies are conducted objectively, they can offer useful baseline data for the evaluation of new practices, techniques and theories. Historically, the value and credibility of single case studies have been debated. When cognitive studies in psychology were out of favour and the objective measurement of overt behaviour was the main source of research records, little attention was formally paid to investigations that concentrated on ONE person rather than on large numbers of people. Relatively few single case studies were accepted for publication. Those that reached the journals did so mainly if a treatment had been shown to be effective. By comparison, many group design studies were published even if the treatment under investigation had not been successful. This led to single case studies being disproportionally represented in the literature.

One major reason for the decline of single case studies was the fact that it was impossible to generalize any results you obtained and many researchers viewed the results from such studies as idiosyncratic. A particular criticism was that because they did not have a universal application, single case studies were somehow unscientific. Bryman (1989: 173) commented however that 'The aim is not to infer the findings from a sample to a population, but to engender patterns and linkages of theoretical importance.' He also emphasized (1989: 175) that 'Case studies provide one of the best arenas in which quantitative and qualitative research can be combined.'

Since behavioural and social scientists have revived their interest in cognitive processes and subjective reports, there has been a marked increase in the number of single case studies reaching publication. It has become 'respectable' to find ways of measuring and analysing what people say, feel and think – all of which can only be taken from their spoken or written reports of their inner reactions. Since they can apply to any of the research designs outlined in this section, the distinction between quantitative measures (counting HOW MANY or HOW OFTEN events happen) and qualitative measures (noting the PERCEIVED and REPORTED experiences of people) is considered in greater detail in Chapter 3.

Group studies

Rather than observing one person in great detail, researchers have collected information about a large number of people, so that the answer to a particular research question could be confirmed. Subsequently, they have analysed their findings, supported by mathematical calculations that provide measures of centrality and dispersion as a means of expressing the common factors revealed by such group studies. It has also been possible to show whether their findings occurred by chance or whether the conditions applied to their group of people had a **significant** bearing on the results. The benefits of studying a lot of people are still rated highly by many people: when we rely on the old adage that there is safety in numbers, we take up the responsibility of being consistent and precise in the way groups are selected for research observation. We must also turn to statistical analysis to find appropriate ways of telling other people about our findings. Statistical analysis and interpretation are discussed more fully in Chapter 5.

2.3 SUBJECT SELECTION

People who agree to be involved in a research project are known as **subjects**, often abbreviated to Ss.

Before we begin recruiting subjects for any research project, it is important to define the group which is to be studied. Is it to be, for example:

- anyone who has a clinical diagnosis of multiple sclerosis (MS)?
- anyone with a diagnosis of MS and who is under 30?
- anyone with MS who is in full-time employment?

Obviously the exact definition of this group will be determined by the idea or hypothesis you want to test. It may be helpful to write down a description of the group of people you wish to study in order to clarify your thoughts.

From the point of view of research, the ideal method for testing your idea would be to include in the investigation the **entire study population** (that you have just defined). However, this would usually be impractical (and you would be bound to miss a hermit living in retreat) so it is necessary to choose a **representative sample**. The important word here is 'representative': other researchers must be able to see that the results you obtain could also be obtained from any person who has the condition or problem you are studying. Consequently your findings could be generalized to any individual with similar problems. A representative group is found by SAMPLING: Burns and Grove (1987: 206) make a succinct comment that:

> Sampling theory was developed to mathematically determine the most effective way of acquiring a sample that would accurately reflect the population under study.

2.3.1 Randomization

A representative sample may be found by taking prospective subjects CONSECUTIVELY or RANDOMLY from a list. A list used in this way is known as the SAMPLING FRAME.

Consecutive sample

A consecutive sample is made by taking the number of patients you decide to use from a list in the order in which they appear. You can decide to start at the beginning, the middle or the end of the list but thereafter you must take names as they are recorded. Examples of lists may be records of hospital admissions, ward admissions, clients referred to social services or specialized lists such as stroke registers.

Although taking a sample in this way may be representative, it may not. For example, if you use the GP list in a middle-class residential area, the results obtained may not be applicable to a poorer area of the city or to a rural community. Similarly, if you survey the number of people who have had contact with social services from the list of a GP with a predominantly elderly patient group, the results may not be applicable to other areas, so your results may be biased.

Random sample

In sampling by random selection all individuals have an equal chance of being chosen. Notice that 'random' does not mean haphazard. The aim of randomization is both to eliminate bias and to be seen to eliminate bias.

There are several types of random sampling.

Simple random sampling

Randomization can be done simply by putting the names of all prospective subjects in a hat and picking out the number required for the study. Equally you could put names on a set of cards, shuffle and deal out the number required. However, it may be easier and less time-consuming to use a table of random numbers (which can be found at the back of most good statistics books) or by requesting a computer to generate random numbers. Once you have made a start with one of these methods, the next task is to decide how you wish to allocate the pool of randomly selected people. This might be by putting them into TWO groups:

1. All even numbers will receive treatment/will be followed up/will have active input.
2. All odd numbers will receive no treatment/will not be followed up/will receive a placebo.

For THREE groups, you might make rules like these:

- exclude all numbers with a 0
- 1, 4, 7 will receive treatment or intervention
- 2, 5, 8 will receive a placebo
- 3, 6, 9 will receive no treatment or intervention.

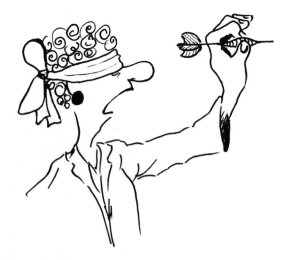

Figure 2.1 Random sample.

Now open at a table of random numbers, select a column and go down the figures. The subject is allocated to a group on the basis of the last figure given. For example:

    53872 – 2
    04226 – 6
    28666 – 6
    63817 – 7
    22359 – 9

In a two group trial, as outlined above, the allocation would be:

    – 2 (even number) treatment
    – 6 (even number) treatment
    – 6 (even number) treatment
    – 7 (odd number) no treatment
    – 9 (odd number) no treatment

If this information is not going to be used immediately, each result should be placed in a numbered, sealed envelope. When you come to subject 35 in your study, for example, open the envelope in front of a witness. In this way others can see that the trial is unbiased: you would obviously have been unable to remember the original allocations for treatment and no treatment and consequently would not have arranged for a fitter patient to draw the treatment group or vice versa.

Block selection
When you are conducting a research project it may be preferable to avoid long periods of comparative inactivity and others in which you are rushing around. This situation may occur in randomization where you could draw the first subjects all for treatment. Apart from the obvious pressure, you may also be unable to give all the subjects the quality of treatment and amount of time you anticipated. Consequently the overall results of the study could be affected. It might therefore be appropriate to consider RESTRICTED RANDOMIZATION by allocating subjects in blocks (Bourke and McGilvray, 1975). This is also known as SEQUENTIAL SAMPLING.

Let us say that we wanted to conduct a trial using 100 subjects, 50 of whom will receive treatment, 50 of whom will not. If we used random tables alone to allocate subjects there would be a risk that we could find that of the first 20 subjects, 18 drew treatment and two drew no treatment. By allocating subjects in blocks of ten we would overcome this difficulty: we would know that in every block of ten subjects drawn, five would be for treatment and five would be controls (no treatment). In order to do this, random tables are used as described above. But as soon as five subjects in every ten are drawn for treatment, the next five are allocated to no treatment (or vice versa if you draw for controls with the first five).

Stratified random sampling
In this method of sampling the population being studied is divided into mutually exclusive categories (STRATA). These subpopulations differ with respect to the feature under study and are of interest themselves (Kirkwood, 1988: 169). For example, suppose you wish to compare the effects of treatment A with those of treatment B. Let us also suppose that you know that sex influences the success of the treatment and that more females are available than males. In order to stratify the sample, you would take 50% of the women and 50% of the men:

Number of females = 70, so 50% of 70 = 35
Number of males = 30, so 50% of 30 = 15

If you do not do this, you could end up with a sampling frame consisting of 40 women and ten men. The results could potentially reflect a male/female influence and not the effect of the treatments. After the subgroups have been identified, a simple random sample can be taken from each stratum.

Cluster sampling
Cluster sampling is used when it would be financially impractical or difficult to collect data. For example, suppose we wished to conduct a study to find out about the attitudes of amputees to Disablement Service Centres (DSCs) throughout the UK. If we used simple random selection we could have a sample that was scattered over an enormous geographical area. Such a study would clearly be impossible to finance and difficult to carry out.

In cluster sampling, groups of the population are selected from the whole (these groups are known thereafter as 'clusters'). Subjects can then be taken from the clusters on a random basis. For example, in the above study, all the DSCs in the UK could be listed (the sampling frame) and several could be selected at random. Once these DSCs have been identified, an agreed number of amputees could be drawn at random from the clients of each chosen DSC.

We might find another example where instead of selecting 10% of the patients registered with all the GPs in a city, we decided to list every practice, select a number of these at random and then make up a cluster sample from the chosen lists. However, although cluster sampling is of great practical importance in a large research project, it has one clear disadvantage. The clusters used in a study may be idiosyncratic and this may lead to bias in the results obtained. Interpretation of results must be cautious when an investigation depends on cluster samples as there is no assurance that all the clusters, taken together, will represent the entire population in a credible way. An interesting paper by Wartenberg and Greenberg (1990) presents a discussion of some important considerations we should make when we are using cluster methods.

Non-random/non-representative selection

Convenience sampling

Convenience sampling is also known as 'haphazard' sampling. Many researchers do not consider it to be an acceptable form of random sampling at all, because essentially any subjects available are recruited for the study in hand. This might be classes of students, a ward of patients, a group of staff: anyone within reach. Unfortunately such a group may not be representative of any other larger population or of the situation being studied. For example, imagine you used this method to study the conditions of patients treated in an out patients' language therapy programme. If you chose to interview patients treated on a day reserved for stroke patients, your results would be misleading.

It is also thought that subjects who volunteer to take part in studies may introduce 'an insidious form of sampling bias' (Spry *et al.*, 1989). That is to say, there may be something different about those individuals who volunteer to participate, those who are paid for it or who are asked to participate in it. Despite all these reservations, where research resources are limited, particularly when time is short, convenience sampling does have a place, especially in a preliminary investigation or a pilot study.

2.3.2 Number of subjects

In order to decide on the number of subjects you need for your research you must first consider the number of people who would be available and the research design to be used. If your population of interest consists of patients with Guillain-Barré Syndrome you will obviously recruit fewer subjects than if you decide to study people with Colles' fractures.

The availability of subjects is not only dependent on clinical incidence or prevalence. Other factors must be taken into account such as the time of year, the weather, the location, hospital policies and concentration of other research in the field. For example, it would be preferable to conduct an investigation of recovery after Colles' fracture in the winter months than in the middle of the summer when the incidence of this fracture is considerably lower.

Next, we should consider that the number of subjects needed can **depend on the design** of the study.

*Related design (also known as **same subject** and **within subject**)*

In such a study, ONE group of subjects is tested on two or more occasions, for example, before and after treatment, and then followed up at three-month and six-month intervals after discharge from hospital.

It is possible for the group to be exposed to all the conditions available (such as treatment and no treatment) and comparisons can be made between the results obtained. The main advantage of using this design is that individual characteristics are eliminated as they are evened out overall. For example, the subject with a memory problem will influence the results in both conditions. However, there are some disadvantages that need to be considered. Suppose we decided to use a questionnaire to ask patients whether they preferred to be treated beside their beds (on the ward) or in the physiotherapy department. The results could be influenced by ORDER EFFECTS: that is, if all the subjects were treated at first in the ward and subsequently in the department, the results might illustrate their satisfaction with that regime. This would need to be adjusted by COUNTERBALANCING: half the subjects could receive treatment at the bedside first (condition A) followed by treatment in the department (condition B) while the other half could have condition B followed by condition A. This would eliminate the possible confounding effects of a constant sequence of treatment/no treatment conditions. It would also address potential problems of:

1. PRACTICE EFFECT: subjects do better on any second questionnaire or test (regardless of the order of treatment) because they have had practice in completing it.
2. FATIGUE EFFECT: subjects do worse on any second questionnaire or test (again regardless of the order of treatment) because they are tired or have less enthusiasm.

If subjects are randomized into this type of design, it is known as a CROSSOVER DESIGN. Remember there are two or more groups of subjects and all groups have the opportunity of receiving the available conditions (treatments). For example, suppose we wanted to find out if patients preferred coming to Out Patients Department (OPD) in an ambulance or in a hospital car. We would:

• randomly select a group of patients

• start half on travelling by ambulance and half on travelling by car

• change the groups over after an agreed time period (Fig. 2.2).

*Unrelated design (**different subject** and **between subject**)*

In this type of study two or more different groups of subjects are tested, for example:

• treatment and no-treatment groups

• placebo and treatment groups

• control, placebo and treatment groups.

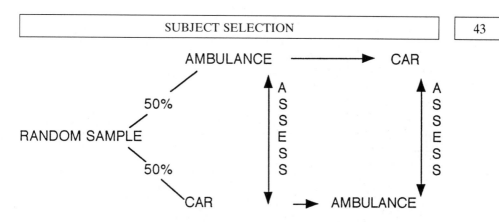

Figure 2.2 Example of a counterbalanced study.

Comparisons are made between the results obtained and conclusions are drawn. This type of design is valuable in situations where it would be impossible to use just one group. For example, in a study comparing the differences in compliance in treatment between men and women, subjects could not be in the same group as they are either male or female. Thus it would be necessary to have at least two groups.

In some situations there is a danger of contamination between groups, or sharing of information. Suppose we taught a group of patients who had had a total hip replacement (THR) some precautions to take while getting dressed in order to eliminate the risk of dislocation. What would happen when we stopped treatment? Would the patients forget everything they had been taught and revert to their pretreatment level of knowledge? The information they had learned would affect the results in the control situation unless a crossover design or, preferably, a two-group design was used.

There is an obvious limitation to the different subject design, namely that the peculiarities of individual subjects will influence the results. Thus a subject with a memory problem will affect the overall performance of her group. This problem can be reduced if you RANDOMIZE subjects into each group, although this is not foolproof. An alternative solution is introduced in the next section.

Matched pairs design

This type of design addresses all the problems mentioned in describing the previous two designs. Basically each subject is matched with a 'twin' and the pair are then randomized into the two groups (treatment and no-treatment). Suppose our study wanted to compare the length of hospital stay for subjects who had had a fractured neck of femur and those who had had a fractured humerus. A one-group design could not be used as people would be unlikely to have both injuries on separate occasions. A two-group design could be used but the two groups of subjects would probably be different. Fractures of the neck of the femur are more common in the elderly and occur more often in the winter months. Consequently, if we just took two groups, we might find that the length of hospital stay was affected by factors other than the injury. We would have to allow for age, speed of healing and whether the patient has someone else living in her home. It would be better to match each subject as closely as possible with someone else. In such a design, the characteristics that might influence results are identified, for example, age, IQ, sex, general health, marital status and home circumstances. These are probably the main confounding variables. Two people are then matched for these factors and allocated randomly to the two conditions (treatment or no-treatment) to be studied. Their performances are then compared in the analysis.

The difficulties of this design are obvious. It is very difficult to really match subjects: is a subject of 40 a suitable 'match' for someone of 35? Moreover, if one subject withdraws from the study, you have effectively lost the results from two people. At this point, it is worth noting that, for the purpose of statistical analysis, matched pairs designs are treated as **related** designs. For example, Reid and Drake (1990) studied nine cerebral palsied children who had spastic diplegia. These children were matched for age and sex with normal children. Reid and Drake found that the disabled children had significantly lower scores in specific perceptual assessments, particularly those for evaluating visual perception.

Management and allocation of subjects

Blind allocation
It is known that those who assess the effects of treatment or no treatment can be influenced by knowing the group to which subjects have been allocated. Assessors, who are often colleagues of the people carrying out the research, can unwittingly tend to be more positive when they are awarding scores to those receiving treatment. Thus it is now common practice to keep assessors in the dark ('blind') as to which group subjects are from. For example, an assessor testing the activities of daily living (ADL) performance of subjects six months after discharge from hospital would not be told who had received follow-up visits at home and who had not.

Double blind allocation
In this type of study neither the researcher nor the assessor is aware of which treatment the subjects have received. Double blind trials are commonly used by doctors, for instance, where neither the doctor giving

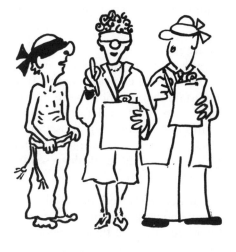

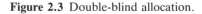

O' Yes 1 see what you mean

Figure 2.3 Double-blind allocation.

the tablet nor the doctor assessing the subject knows who is receiving the medication in the trial or who is taking the placebo. Similar trials may be used in therapy but there are strong opinions on the ethics of withholding treatment. It is also difficult to design activities that have true placebo status.

A prospective and double blind trial in physiotherapy was carried out by Blowman *et al.* (1991). The subjects were patients with stress incontinence who were being treated with pelvic floor exercises. These subjects were allocated on a random basis to two groups; one was given neurotrophic stimulation (NTS) and the other placebo stimulation. Neither the assessors nor the physiotherapist dealing with the pelvic floor exercises knew which group individual subjects belonged to. Results showed that there was a greater effect of pelvic floor exercises when patients were also given NTS.

Sampling and the statistical POWER *of a study*

The power of a study has been defined as 'the probability of rejecting the null hypothesis when it should be rejected' (Bausell, 1986). Put in more simple terms, it is the probability of rejecting the null hypothesis when it cannot be supported. If a study has a low statistical power, the probability of concluding that there is no statistical difference between samples, when a difference does exist, is increased. This is known as a Type II error and is a pessimistic error (Greene and d'Oliveira, 1981: 29).

There are three main reasons why a study can be described as lacking in power:

- Too few subjects were used
  Altman (1982) suggests that many studies are too small to have a reasonable chance of detecting clinical benefits. If a limited number of patients is used, important therapeutic benefits may not be demonstrated because the sample is too small to detect any significance that might occur. Where the differences between groups anticipated is small, large numbers of subjects are needed. If the sample size planned for a study is too small to illustrate a significant level, the researcher should question the decision to conduct the study.

- The most precise statistical tests were not used
  Some statistical tests demonstrate significance more readily than others. A one-tailed test is more powerful than a two-tailed test, a parametric test is more powerful than a non-parametric test (see Chapter 5).

- The data collection and/or the analysis was not carried out carefully
  For more details on estimating the power of a study, see Cohen (1977), Burns and Grove (1987: 480–3) and Bourke and McGilvray (1975: 86–7, 313–14). There is also an interesting article by Gore (1981) which examines the sizes of clinical trials with an emphasis on power.

2.3.3 Subject exclusions

Exclusions from a research study must be defined initially. It is essential that only those subjects who would bias the sample or who would contribute no relevant information are excluded. There must be sound reasons for deciding to exclude a group of individuals from a study. The exclusions will be different for each study depending on the question to be answered. For example, it would be appropriate to exclude blind people from a study of hemianopia after a cerebrovascular accident (CVA) but not from a study on dressing difficulties after CVA.

2.3.4 Non-respondents

Information should ideally be collected on non-respondents: that is, those who fail to attend for interview or do not return questionnaires. They should not merely be 'written off' and no longer considered. It may be that as a group they differ in some way from the rest of the sample. They may represent an important subgroup of special interest. When people do not respond, they may:

- have died
- have moved

- have had less education and be unable to understand or complete the questionnaire
- not speak English
- be socially deprived and unable to attend the interview
- be very disabled and unable to post their questionnaire or use the taxi you have sent to bring them to the interview you had planned.

It is therefore worth while contacting these individuals to see if they are having particular problems in responding or if they merely need a reminder. One method is to send stamped addressed envelopes to those who have not replied, supplying them with another questionnaire or a new date for an interview. Spry *et al.* (1989) found that speaking to people on the telephone was the most effective way to follow up the non-respondents. Remember that although it is sound research to check up on why some people do not respond, they must not be pressurised into participating (see Ethical considerations, section 1.3).

<table>
<tr><td>**3**</td><td colspan="2">**Methods and tools of investigation**</td></tr>
</table>

3.1 INTRODUCTION

In Chapter 2, we explored the general designs that can be used in any investigation. We now need to consider a range of methods in detail, before selecting the ones that will suit the character of your project. Research in health settings usually depends on the methods of the social sciences, particularly because the work is carried out with people and can rarely be controlled in the exact way that experiments can be governed within pure science. In health or social services, the researcher needs the subjects' informed consent and plans for the investigation have to meet ethical standards. Once your project has been fully planned, a proposal (or protocol) has to be submitted to the ethical committee whose jurisdiction covers the population from which you are planning to invite participants. Provided that the ethical committee is convinced that your study will have no detrimental effect on the people who will be acting as your subjects, it is usual for approval to be given. This whole topic is considered further by Carr (1991) who gives an excellent résumé of ethical considerations.

It would not be feasible in this introductory book to give an exhaustive account of the whole range of research methods but this chapter discusses some of the methods most commonly used by therapists. None of them carries a complete recipe for your research and all of them have to be used within a framework that you, as the researcher, sets up and adheres to. The general methods can be interpreted and varied to match your research needs, but once the 'rules' have been set for any project they must not be altered **within** the study. For example, you can decide to collect measurements from three groups of people, dividing them on the basis of their employment and age into Group A: 20–25-year-olds, Group B: 40–45-year-olds and Group C: 60–65-year-olds. It would not be acceptable after you have been working on your study for six months to change Group C to include some people aged 56–59 because you are having difficulty in finding enough people who are still employed in the original age band.

The methods to be considered in the sections that follow are characterized as:

3.1 Observation
3.2 Survey: postal questionnaires
               interviews
               telephone interviews
3.3 Analysis of existing records
3.4 Clinical trials
3.5 Single subject experiments/studies

3.2 OBSERVATION

Observation has been defined by *The Oxford Dictionary* as both the 'faculty of taking notice' and 'accurate watching and noting of phenomena as they occur in nature'. It is used in the research context to describe a method in which 'behaviour or an event, where there are no constraints on what occurs, is recorded directly in the specific setting in which it happens and is observed in the environmental context within which it actually occurs' (Cormack, 1984: 90). It is a direct method of collecting information and indicates what subjects actually do as opposed to what we think they do or what they say they do.

Observations can be used in situations where subjects, such as young children, would be unable to answer questions or where there is no relevant tool for obtaining the information needed. Descriptions are important for clarifying practice and this in turn may provide a useful baseline from which an area can be explored more fully by using other research methods or by developing questionnaires. Carr (1991: 93) notes that 'a wealth of otherwise unobtainable data awaits those willing to explore its use'.

Many people view observation in research as an easy technique – which it is not. The rigorous observation of a formal investigation requires people to avoid bias and to be as objective as possible. The ability to learn and be faithful to such skills has profound professional implications. To use observation successfully, it must be carefully planned; you cannot amble into a situation hoping to record anything you see happening. First, you must have a clear statement of what outcome is anticipated or what specific area you are looking at. Before beginning you must:

1. **Define the behaviour in which you are interested**
   For example, in a study by Gee (1991) who wanted to research the interpersonal contact behaviours of subjects, the therapist first had to

identify the behaviours – 'contact indicators' – (eye contact, facial expression) and 'withdrawal behaviours' – (crying, talking in nonsense words), before allocating scores.

2. **Attempt to reduce or to minimize the observer's influence on the situation**

People react differently from normal when they are being studied (for example, they may work harder, be more polite or curb anti-social behaviour). Thus the presence of the observer may alter the true situation. Consequently allowances must be made for this and the subjects must be given time to 'forget about' the observer. If you wish to collect the data by direct observation, you must decide on the level of involvement of the observer. Gold (1958) states that this ranges from acting as a 'complete participant' to being a 'complete observer'. In the former, the researcher observes and is involved in the research situation, while in the latter she observes without becoming integrated into the situation. As an alternative, the observer can be on one side of a two-way mirror between her room and the area being watched. This allows a subject or a group of subjects to be under observation without any intrusion on the behaviours and interactions going on. Although the observer is in a separate room, it is still necessary for the subjects to agree to participate in the study.

Observation may also be carried out by using a video recorder: once again, time must be given for the subjects to become used to the camera. It is important to emphasize that the video recorder should not be sneaked in; subjects must be aware that they are being filmed. However, people tend to forget about the presence of a video camera more quickly than they do the presence of a human observer. Carr (1991) makes some interesting points about the choice between 'live' and video observation and this paper is well worth reading if you are unsure about the advantages and disadvantages of each. Ultimately the context of the situation will determine the most satisfactory method of observation.

3. **Decide on the method of scoring**

Scoring may be done live or from a video recording. Pen and paper checklists, rating scales or more advanced digital keyboards may be used. Details of rating scales are discussed in Chapter 4. For further information about digital keyboards, see Sackett (1979).

If the information recorded is to be used for statistical analysis, the way it has been collected must be seen to be reliable and valid. You will have to decide whether to use an observation period of a constant time or whether to take samples at intervals. The sampling method records only behaviour that occurs during randomly selected periods of time and uses these records in the subsequent analysis (see Chapter 2 for an explanation of the principles of sampling). Decisions must also be made about the venue(s) that are to be used for observation periods. It is important that similar surroundings are available for all observation sessions, with an agreed minimum of resources (equipment, furniture, staff and other specified facilities).

When scoring, it is important that a behaviour is not missed because the observer is busy recording a previous behaviour. It is also essential that everything that is wanted can be recorded; 'each response must be capable of discrimination by the observer so that it can be measured' (Cormack, 1984: 92). Decisions must be made on how to quantify observations; does something occur? If it does occur, what is the frequency? When and where does it occur? (that is, what is the relationship of the observed behaviour to other events?) Is there a regular sequence of events?

All observers involved in the study must record information in the same way. As Hilgard, Atkinson and Atkinson (1979: 18) rightly comment, 'Investigators must be trained to observe and record accurately in order to avoid projecting their own wishes or biases onto what they report.' Thus there should be intra- and inter-rater reliability. Remember, high inter-rater agreement does not of itself mean that the records are reliable: it is a **necessary** but not a **sufficient** condition of reliability (see Chapter 2 for information on reliability).

Systems and strategies for recording information need to be checked for their realistic use. Particularly where a study is based on observing qualitative features, there is a tendency to attempt to record everything in a situation. If the observer tries to describe all events in detail rather than allocating a score at the time, this becomes a very time-consuming process. The initial written notes must then be transcribed, usually resulting in a long and detailed account that has to be studied and scored. Another problem with written records, as well as with using set scoring indicators, is that data can be lost by reducing complex situations to fit into agreed categories (Carr, 1991: 89). A video recording has the clear advantage that the action can be revisited, allowing several opportunities to make sure that no important elements have been missed but without the intervening, potentially selective, task of written description. However, it is wise to consider all aspects of the video-recording process before adopting it. There are advantages and disadvantages, some of which are indicated below.

Advantages of using video recording:

- filming can be carried out in the natural setting of the events being studied

- there are few costs to be met, except for the cost of the video tape

- it can be used with subjects who cannot be interviewed directly

- non-verbal behaviours can be captured accurately for later analysis.

Disadvantages of using video recording:

- the 'camera man' needs time and experience to make sure that behaviours and events are shot from suitable angles

- preparation of equipment and conditions for filming is time-consuming

- analysing the filmed record is a long process.

4. Consider how to analyse data

It is important that the interpretation of behaviour has a rational base and can be linked where possible to an accepted form of analysis. The type of analysis you choose will interact with the characteristics of the information you decide to collect (your data), as well as with the conditions for collection. Unless you are an expert in statistical management and interpretation of data, you would be wise to discuss with a statistician the possible ways and means of assembling the information you are expecting. This is important so that you record information in a suitable way, you collect ONLY the data you will use and you will be able to tell colleagues and interested others about your work, preferably by publishing a full and lucid report of your study. It is ideal if this discussion with a statistician/adviser can happen before details of your design and methods have been finalized for inclusion in your proposal. Certainly, before any data are collected, you must have a clear plan for managing all the categories of information your project will generate.

3.3 SURVEY

All surveys have flaws, but high-quality surveys make an honest attempt to accomplish their purposes with accurate unbiased questions.

Weisberg and Bowen (1977: 57)

The term 'survey' is defined in *The Oxford Dictionary* as 'the act of examining or inspecting for some specific purpose'. Surveys are used to describe and summarize observations from a group of individuals. They are used for five main purposes (Drummond, 1990):

1. to identify problems in a preliminary study
2. to establish the size or extent of a problem

3. to provide a baseline so that the effects of a subsequent intervention programme can be monitored
4. for the collection of data for audit purposes
5. where the use of a randomized control trial is impossible, for example in a situation where it is impossible to have a control group.

The methods of data collection in a survey include asking questions by face-to-face contact, by post or by telephone. In all these approaches, the value of the research depends to a large extent on the quality of the questions being asked.

Practical considerations in designing questions

Types of question
Questions may be categorised into two main groups: namely 'closed' questions and 'open' questions.

Closed questions A closed question may be defined as one 'which requires the respondent to choose his answer from a given, limited selection' (Bennett and Ritchie, 1975). Subjects are asked to tick a box, circle an answer or fill in an answer taken from a limited number of alternatives, such as:

> What is your present marital status? The answer must be one of the following: single, married, separated, divorced or widowed.

Or:

> Which of the following would you use to rate the treatment you have received from the ward therapist since your admission to this Unit? Choose your answer from: excellent, good, quite good, fair or poor.

Or:

> How often do you have a bath?
>
> every day   _____
>
> twice a week   _____
>
> less than twice a week   _____
>
> never   _____

Or:

> Do you agree or disagree with the following statements?
> I worry about having another heart attack   □ agree□ disagree
> I am trying to increase the amount of exercise I do□ agree□ disagree

Thus responses to closed questions are relatively easy to analyse as they come from a known and limited pool. They are therefore readily coded for analysis by a computer.

Open questions By contrast, no such specific response is suggested in an open question where the respondent 'is allowed to answer freely, in his own words, and his response is recorded in full' (Bennett and Ritchie, 1975). Samples of open questions could be:

> Describe your feelings after you were told that you might never be able to walk again.

Or:

> How do you feel about the treatment you have received from the ward therapists since your admission to this Unit?

Using open questions can encourage the subject to provide more information as the interviewer can probe additional clues and comments more fully. However, in order to compare responses to open questions across a number of subjects, systems for identifying key words or themes must be set up as the first step in the analysis of results.

Content of questions
It is important that you only ask questions that are relevant to the study: questions should not be asked for any other reason, for instance 'in case it might be interesting as a sideline'. You must also recognize that some questions are potentially embarrassing for the subject or will cause distress and upset. There is no easy way to avoid this dilemma. You must be sensitive to the subjects' feelings and phrase your questions accordingly.

On a lighter note, I recommend an extremely amusing paper by Barton (1958) on the subject of phrasing embarrassing questions. Several potential techniques are outlined as methods of obtaining an answer to the question 'Did you kill your wife?' My particular favourites are:

> The casual approach:
> Do you happen to have murdered your wife?

> The 'everybody' approach:
> As you know, many people have been killing their wives these days. Do you happen to have killed yours?

Way of asking questions
Although Barton's paper is very funny, it does make the point that the way you ask questions is important. This applies to potentially sensitive topics and indeed to all areas. The researcher must be careful not to lead the subject in the way questions are phrased. For example:

Don't you think that . . .
Do you not think that abortion is murder?
Don't you think smoking is a disgusting and anti-social habit?

You must be neither approving or disapproving nor show any surprise at the subject's responses.

Similarly you must be careful about the wording of your questions. DO NOT

- ask double-barrelled questions, using 'or' to connect two questions, for example 'Do you prefer treatment at home or in hospital?'

- be ambiguous or vague, for example, 'What do you think of the hospital?' or 'Do you attend regularly?'

- use technical language, for example, 'When did you have your myocardial infarction?'

Boyle (1970) conducted a very interesting study to compare the differences between patients' and doctors' understanding of some relatively common medical terms. The results demonstrated a significant difference between the two groups: the only term they seemed to agree on was 'a good appetite'.

The order in which questions are asked is important. It is usual to ask subjects more administrative questions such as their date of birth and address first. Sensitive questions are usually placed later. Similarly, the context in which questions are asked is important. A person may be unwilling to admit to having a bad cough after admitting to being a smoker, but may admit to both if the same questions are asked in reverse order.

Length of survey
As a rough rule of thumb, there should be no more than 20–25 words in a question and a questionnaire or interview should take no longer than 20–25 minutes to complete. This means that the NUMBER of questions to be asked must be kept as low as possible. You must be sure that every question asked can be justified: that is, the answers to that question are essential to meet the aim of the survey.

Covering letter
All subjects who are approached with regard to participating in a survey should be sent a letter of explanation. Briefly, the letter should outline the purpose of the study, give the name of a contact person and assure confidentiality and anonymity.

Thank you
Last but not least, remember it is important to say thank you to everyone who has helped in the research as your subjects. This may be done orally

or, if finance permits, a letter may be sent. Researchers who take their subjects for granted risk creating a poor reputation for themselves: it is likely to be more difficult to find willing participants for their next project.

3.3.1 Postal questionnaires

A questionnaire is not just a list of questions or a form to be filled out. It is essentially a scientific instrument for measurement and for collection of particular kinds of data.

Oppenheim (1966: 2)

It must be emphasised that questionnaires are often only opinion-naires.

Treece and Treece (1977: 183)

The use of postal questionnaires is probably the most popular method of obtaining information from subjects. Many researchers seem to be under the illusion that they can run up a questionnaire in an evening, have it typed and just send it out. Nothing could be further from the truth. The actual construction, design and layout of a questionnaire is a very skilled craft; proficiency in this skill does not develop overnight.

Considerations

Presentation

- Is the questionnaire typed and laid out neatly?
- Is the colour of the paper appropriate?
- Is the order of questions logical and easy to follow?
- Is the section 'For office use only' clearly designated?

Questions

- Are the questions easy to understand?
- Are any of the questions ambiguous?
- Are the questions worded correctly?

Completion
Is it clear how the questionnaire should be completed? For example:

- Do you tick boxes or circle answers?
- Can you have more than one answer to each question?
- What do you do if there is not enough space to answer a question?
- Who do you ask if you want to verify something?

Return

How do you return the completed questionnaire? For example:

- Is there an envelope provided?
- Do you need a stamp?
- Will someone collect it or do you need to post it?
- Who do you return it to and where are they based?

Advantages of postal questionnaires

- They are relatively inexpensive. Costs can be reduced by using cheaper quality paper and by not enclosing stamped addressed envelopes, although leaving these out may have an adverse effect on the response rate. Moreover, staff do not need to be trained to interview subjects. Imagine the cost if the government relied on interviewing everyone when conducting a national census.
- A large area can be surveyed; there are few geographical limitations to distribution. For example, Beard and Fergusson (1992) conducted a national postal survey of 30 centres in the UK to collect information on non-surgical treatment of anterior cruciate ligament deficiency. Among the results obtained was the fact that only 5% of centres saw patients with such an injury within three months of injury and few centres had a definite treatment protocol. In a further example, Reid (1992) surveyed paediatric occupational therapists working in Canada on their use of hand splints for children with neuromuscular dysfunction. It was found that 50% of those surveyed used only three splints regularly.
- A large number of people can be approached. Compare this with the time, energy and cost involved in surveying 100 individuals by post with that of interviewing them separately.
- Information can be collected quickly. You can be confident that all subjects have received the same information via a standardized package. All subjects are therefore open to the same, if any, researcher bias. Subjects can be more confident that their replies are anonymous when they send information by mail, especially when they do not have to put their name on anything they send. If the study is well-prepared and planned, results should be comparatively straightforward to analyse.

Disadvantages of postal questionnaires

- The response rate with postal questionnaires is recognized as low. If people are interested in the subject, the response is usually between 40% and 60%. However, even when people are interested, response above 80% is rare (Oppenheim, 1966: 34).
- Subjects are not able to ask what a question means. It is only possible to

answer the questions printed on the questionnaire and people may not feel that they have the opportunity to elaborate on topics about which they have strong feelings. This may mean that their answers are superficial and that their individuality is lost.

- There is little chance of setting up rapport with the subject and gaining his confidence and cooperation.
- Postal surveys make the assumption that people are able to complete the questionnaire. However, written responses to printed questions discriminate against people who are blind, illiterate or who have language difficulties. Similarly, people with mobility problems may have difficulty in leaving their homes to post a letter or in getting someone to post it for them.
- You must assume that subjects are honest in their replies.
- Preparation and design of the questionnaire is very time-consuming.
- Postal surveys are susceptible to Acts of God and unpredictable events. They can be affected by such diverse factors as poor weather preventing people from going out to mail their completed questionnaires, postal strikes delaying responses that have been mailed and the unexpected generally.

3.3.2 Interviews

A method of collecting data from a subject face-to-face by asking questions.

Miller and Wilson (1983)

A conversation with a purpose.

Partridge and Barnitt (1986)

Interviews may be used in exploratory work or in descriptive studies. It is generally considered that they produce much richer information than postal questionnaires. Interviews vary with regard to the type of questions asked and the dominance of the interviewer or interviewee. They may be considered in three categories: structured, unstructured and semi-structured interviews.

Structured interviews

The researcher is in control of the content of the dialogue in a structured interview. Questions are prepared in advance and the same wording and order of questions are used with each subject. The researcher should not adapt or elaborate on the questions being asked; no clarification may be offered to subjects who are told to answer in whatever way they interpret the question. However, it is usual to allow the researcher to repeat a question if this is needed. An INTERVIEW SCHEDULE (see Chapter 4) may be used to assist the interviewer. The main advantage of structured interviews is that the results are easier to analyse than those of an unstructured one. This may be at the cost of overlooking valuable information because the interviewer was not in a position to ask further questions which might have revealed such important facts or issues.

Unstructured interviews

In this situation, the interviewee is in control and is encouraged to elaborate and expand on the opinions and feelings mentioned. Such interviews are valuable in exploratory studies or when you are developing research instruments. The format may be UNSTRUCTURED where the interviewer has the freedom to explore any topic as it arises. However, most interviewers have an INTERVIEW GUIDE from which to work. Interviews may be FOCUSED: that is, although the researcher has freedom in each interview to conduct it as it develops, there is a tendency to concentrate on specific topics. Unfortunately there is a risk that all the interviews turn out differently and this makes it difficult to code and process the information obtained. Some investigators argue that this is a strength: their objective is to understand the subject by trying to become immersed in the views of individual respondents. Many anthropology studies have been carried out on this premise.

Semi-structured interviews

As the name suggests, these interviews are a mixture of the two types of interview outlined above. Generally the researcher has a list of specific questions to be asked but is free to pursue the points of interest that arise.

Recording interview data

It is obviously vital to have a valid record of each interview. Records can be made by:

- the interviewer filling up a printed questionnaire
- the interviewer keeping handwritten notes, taken during or immediately after the interview
- a tape recorder
- a video recorder. This has been less common in the past but its use is rapidly increasing.

The decision about which method to use will depend on the preferences of the researcher and subjects, the resources available and the field or area of the research. The method of recording data should offer as little distraction as possible to the person being interviewed.

Preparation for interviews

Environment
This should be private, comfortable and quiet (never compete with the TV). There should be no interruptions: it is wise to ask others not to disturb you and take the telephone off the hook. The same or similar environment should be used for interviewing all your subjects.

Time
Consider the timing of interviews. For example, if you wish to interview patients who have returned to work, it will be difficult if you only offer appointments during your working hours. Also consider how long the interview is likely to take and inform the subject accordingly. You do not want the subject concentrating on the possibility of missing a bus rather than on your interview. Equally you do not want one subject to have a disproportionate amount of time. You will be able to gauge the time needed from conducting pilot studies.

Consistency
There must be consistency between interviews and between interviewers. This can be assessed by testing for inter-rater reliability. It is important to ensure that not only is the content of interviews similar but also that the style is equivalent. Practice sessions (training sessions) should be organized for people who will be conducting interviews and there should be feedback available from pilot interviews. Attention must be paid to the type and range of cues to be given to the people who are being interviewed. Provided that the indicators are agreed by all interviewers and used for all subjects, people may be encouraged by non-verbal means such as making eye contact, head nodding, using gestures and smiling as well as by using standard signal words such as 'good', 'yes and what else?', 'that's fine'.

Sequence of questions
Consideration should be given to the order of presenting subject matter. It is usual to begin with safe questions, such as those about the length of time in hospital or marital status. Move on to more sensitive subjects later.

Recording interview data
The interviewer(s) should be familiar with the agreed method of recording the data. Any abbreviations or 'short cuts' which can speed up the recording process must be consistent, without ambiguity and used by everyone working on the project. Sufficient practice in using the recording system should be given so that the interviewer is not preoccupied with noting responses during the interview. It is also important for each

interviewer to know how to operate any equipment she has to use, such as a tape recorder.

Dress and appearance
This should be appropriate for the situation and environment. Choice of dress is largely a matter of sensitivity and commonsense. Remember that inappropriate dress may alter the subjects' willingness to talk to you. You are likely to set up immediate barriers if you choose to wear an expensive suit when talking to teenagers at a drug abuse clinic or ripped jeans when interviewing an elderly population in an exclusive rest home.

Guidelines for conducting an interview

> There is more to being a good interviewer than asking the questions you want to have answered.
>
> Breakwell (1990: 1)

1. Introduce yourself. Explain the purpose of the interview and make sure that the interviewee (subject) has already given consent to take part in the study.
2. Assure each subject that everything mentioned in the interview will be treated with confidentiality and will be anonymous.
3. Try to establish RAPPORT with the subject.
4. Keep the aim of the study in the forefront, particularly when an unstructured interview is in progress.
5. Remember that much information is available without the need to ask questions, for example about sex, approximate age, colouring.
6. Respect the subjects' right to leave some questions unanswered. Do not oblige people to answer a question if they do not want to do so. Subjects should not feel pressurized in any way: remember, they have volunteered to assist you and you do not want to lose their cooperation.
7. When you are asking questions, AVOID:

   ● being aggressive

   ● being approving or disapproving or surprised

   ● asking double-barrelled questions which give an 'either . . . or' option, for example, 'Do you prefer treatment at home or in hospital?'

   ● being vague or asking ambiguous questions

   ● using technical language

   ● using leading phrases.

Check again on the practical considerations given earlier in this chapter at section 3.3.

Advantages of interviews

> The greatest advantage of the interview in the hands of a skilled interviewer is its flexibility.
>
> Oppenheim (1966: 31)

- Both parties can repeat information or ask for clarification so that there is less chance of misunderstandings.

- In semi-structured and unstructured interviews, the researcher can follow up relevant lines by asking subjects to elaborate on their response. Consequently more detailed information can be collected.

- There is greater flexibility than in using a postal questionnaire.

- Some people find it easier to express themselves by talking than by writing.

- Information can be provided by those who may be excluded from replying to a postal questionnaire, for example, those who cannot read or write, or those who are unable to post a letter.

- The interviewer has the opportunity to establish rapport with the subject. This may improve their cooperation and willingness to answer questions.

- Subjects who attend an interview will answer some questions, so the response rate will be higher and the sample more representative than in an equivalent postal questionnaire, for which the proportion of questionnaires returned is likely to be low.

Disadvantages of interviews

- The time involved in actually interviewing subjects, transcribing interviews and processing data is great. Compare the work involved in interviewing 50 subjects with that of sending out 50 postal questionnaires.
- The expense of staff time, travel costs (for you or the subjects) and administrative costs must all be considered and may well be greater than those involved in alternative ways of data collection.
- Interviews need to be conducted by a skilled interviewer.
- Recording the information obtained can be difficult. There can be problems in reading rushed notes, individual abbreviations and 'short cuts' to expressing what was observed and in transcribing tape

recordings. There are also problems in comparing results obtained from different interviewers, no matter how rigid the interview structure.

- Information may be difficult to code and analyse. For example, you may realize that a subject is being sarcastic in a particular comment but be unable to code that impression as well as the actual words they used.
- Although subjects may be assured of anonymity by the researcher, they may still feel threatened and inhibited.
- The researcher must assume that the subject replies honestly.
- There are opportunities for interviewer bias.

Biased questions are questions that make one response more likely than another, regardless of the respondent's opinion.

Weisberg and Bowen (1977: 45)

Other problem areas include:

Acquiescence
The subject answers 'Yes' to every question asked.

Conforming
Subjects try to conform to the ideas of the interviewer, for example, telling a speech and language therapist that speech therapy was the most important aspect of their rehabilitation programme.

Experimenter bias effect
The interviewer, either consciously or not, uses subtle influences (such as voice inflections, pausing at certain phrases) to lead the subject to make responses that confirm the hypothesis.

Halo effect
This refers to the tendency of the interviewer to bias her judgement of the interviewee on the basis of one feature. This then influences her interpretation of other aspects of the interview. The bias can be either positive or negative. Although it is usually a positive bias, both are equally misleading. If we agree with the opinions of the person we are interviewing, we are more likely to see other responses in a positive way: for example, the interviewer may decide that the prettiest subject is also the most intelligent.

Hawthorne effect
In this situation, extra attention from the interviewer affects the outcome. It is recognized that the mere fact that someone is involved in an investigation affects their performance. This effect was first described by Simon in 1969. A group conducting research at the Hawthorne plant of the

Western Electric Company found that, regardless of the working conditions, productivity increased. The reason was that workers knew they were being observed so they worked harder.

Stereotype

This describes the tendency to over-generalize. We assume that every member of a group has particular characteristics, for example, a woman wearing flat brogues and pearls is from the middle class.

Prestige bias

This refers to the desire of the subjects to please the interviewer and to be seen in a better light, for example, the subjects deny ever forgetting to wash their hands after using the toilet.

Examples of interview-based research

Cheng and Rogers (1989) interviewed ten men who had sustained severe burns. The interviews were held in the year after their rehabilitation. The aim of the study was to examine their perceptions of the impact of receiving such injuries.

N.A. Roberts (1990) carried out a prospective study which followed up a random sample of 100 patients seen in an accident and emergency unit. Subjects were interviewed in their own homes, using a questionnaire. The study concluded that although many of the injuries sustained would only be classified as minor, they had major implications for the functional abilities for a number of patients. Moreover, it found that many of the people interviewed would not have coped without the support of their family and friends.

3.3.3 Telephone interviews

At present there is a growing interest in the use of telephone interviews for research purposes. There seems great potential in the idea of contacting large numbers of subjects and receiving information immediately. Interviews could be conducted for use in large multicentre studies or in studies where direct assessment is unrealistic or too expensive. However, some people are suspicious of answering questions over the telephone and are nervous that you are really trying to sell them double glazing. This problem may be alleviated by sending letters out to subjects before you call them so that they are expecting to hear from you. The obvious disadvantage of this is the additional cost involved in mailing the letters.

Telephone interviewing does have great potential as a method of collecting information from other professionals. Shinar *et al.* (1987)

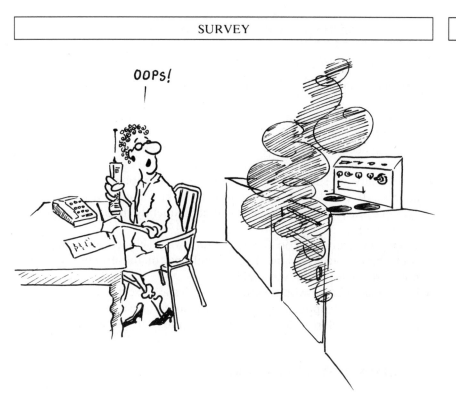

Figure 3.1 Telephone interviews.

examined the validity of an Activities of Daily Living scale administered by telephone interview by comparing the results with those obtained by observation of actual performance. They found that they could obtain a valid ADL assessment from telephone interviews conducted by well-trained professionals. However the authors note that 'Care should be taken to assure that telephone interviews are not with a sample that may be biased in any way that would directly affect scoring on the verbal responses versus performance.'

Advantages of telephone surveys

- Reliability. Potentially they are just as reliable as collecting data in face-to-face interviews.
- Numbers. Large numbers of people can be contacted.
- Area. A large geographical area can be surveyed.
- Speed. Information can be collected quickly.
- Clarity. Questions can be clarified immediately.
- Acceptability. Telephone interviewing may be more acceptable to some subjects than face-to-face questioning (Breakwell, 1990: 84).

Disadvantages of telephone surveys

- Expense. Using a telephone is more expensive than using the postal service.
- Inconvenience. You may have to call at different times to get the person you want in the house or office.
- Training needs. Assessors need to be well-trained and, where more than one is involved, inter-rater reliability needs to be established.
- Availability of subjects. Fewer people have a phone than have an address. It could be said therefore that the sample was biased (for example, richer, more disabled and consequently in greater need of a telephone).
- Competing activity. You cannot be sure what subjects are doing: they could be distracted by the TV, a family pet or the ironing. Similarly, non-verbal cues are not available.
- Exclusions. People with hearing difficulties are excluded.
- Dependence on spoken cues. Complex closed questions are difficult to answer, particularly when a number of options are available.

3.4 ANALYSIS OF EXISTING RECORDS

Records can provide a rich source of information for the researcher. The term 'records' can apply to general administrative information kept on patients and to specific records such as medical notes and reports kept by individual departments. Usually the latter type of records are needed by the therapist conducting a research project.

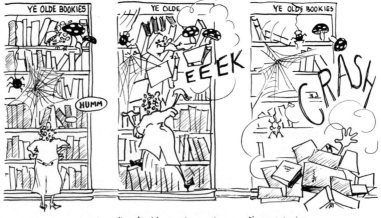

Searching through old records can be very time consuming

Figure 3.2 Analysis of existing records.

Records can be used RETROSPECTIVELY as a source of information or they can be kept for specific research purposes (PROSPECTIVELY). In the latter, if staff are being asked to keep additional information beyond their normal job requirements, forms for data collection should be as simple and easy as possible to complete. In a situation where many staff are filling in such forms, instructions and guidelines must be available to assist them.

The first step in consulting past records is usually to seek permission to do so. The consultant who is in charge of a patient should be approached for their consent to look at his/her medical records. Similarly, the head of the appropriate department must be asked for consent to the records and reports in her department being read. It is always advisable to put your requests into a letter which should outline the purpose of the study and guarantee confidentiality and anonymity. It may also be appropriate to offer a copy of the final research report to the consultant or head of department involved. It is not a good idea to approach someone in the corridor, regardless of how well you know them, and ask for permission to conduct such a study. Formal written requests should always be made and copies of these letters and their replies should be filed with your research papers.

Remember that the people you approach are more likely to give their consent if they are assured that the department can anticipate minimal disruption to its day-to-day running. If staff believe that you will be constantly needing help to find or interpret something, unshelving rows of neatly filed records, or being an obstacle in the middle of a busy office, they are likely to refuse. So it is important to ensure that you can guarantee that this will not happen or that you have made some plans to minimize disruption, for example, by arranging to have set times for asking staff about queries instead of bothering them every few minutes.

A final point to remember: always keep the aim of your study to the forefront of your mind. It is very easy to get waylaid by interesting facts and figures when you are reading old records. This may be interesting from a personal point of view but it is likely to do nothing for the study in hand. It is a good idea to have a checklist, questionnaire or other research tool to enable you to focus on your research.

Advantages and disadvantages of using existing records

Advantages

1. It is a relatively inexpensive method of collecting information. For example, records in each department tend to be stored in one area, thus reducing your costs and travel time.
2. Data are already available.

3. Data may be available over several years and thus an overall perspective can be gauged on each subject or situation.
4. Information may be available from a number of sources so that it may be possible to collect a profile of the multidisciplinary service.
5. Information should be unbiased, particularly if the people who kept the records did not anticipate them being used for research purposes.

Disadvantages

1. Information such as date of birth, addresses, marital status or diagnosis may be inadequate, inaccurate or incomplete. Such partial or inaccurate information may be passed on when therapists refer patients to each other, leading to duplication of mistakes. This makes it difficult to cross-check accurately.
2. Information may be missing from notes: records may be lost, misfiled or destroyed.
3. Consulting records is a very time-consuming activity and (dare I say it?) often very tedious.
4. Help may be needed from others in the department to find and interpret old records.
5. Important information needs to be cross-referenced with other sources either internally (using other records) or externally (referring to the subjects involved, or to census material).
6. Information may be subjective. It may be difficult to collect information on the people who actually recorded this information, their experience or the prevailing situation. So there may be unknown personal bias.
7. Disturbance to departmental routine. The researcher who sits on the floor of a busy office surrounded by stacks of files never endears herself or her study to the other staff.
8. Dust! Any researcher who has ever conducted a study based on past records will realize that the older the records, the greater the volume of dust there is to overcome.

Some of these advantages and disadvantages can be seen in the work of Anderson, Llewellyn and Bell (1991) who undertook an audit of occupational therapy records, based on material and notes about adults with developmental difficulties. They found that, although records did exist, the majority varied in adequacy of standardization. This finding emphasized that the diversity of the methods and content of records can make it difficult to draw any conclusions of a general nature.

Prospective studies based on purpose-kept records

In addition to the listed advantages and disadvantages of analysing past records, it is as well to note that **prospective** studies themselves can induce changes in practice. Because a prospective study calls for additional or different information to be collected in some areas, this is likely to influence the way in which the staff record all treatments. By altering the emphasis of observations, it may also bring in some changes that affect service routines and lead to general modifications in practice. If this happens, it is not a question of evaluating the changes themselves but of being aware that the environment and situation is different from the one in which you originally set up your study. It would be necessary to analyse and report the changes in practice when you are considering the limitations and general biases of your study.

Although the staff in each service or treatment unit are confronted by particular research questions, most departments base their projections for future manpower and resource on analysis of the numbers of referrals, types of disorders, reasons for admissions, rate of discharges and costs of care. Most of these details can be taken from records kept during the current or preceding years. In a climate of resource limitations and obligation to provide efficient care, there is a pressing need to maintain accurate records and to analyse these regularly and exactly.

Let us assume that the social services of a local authority has to decide the budget for its speech and language therapy department. It needs evidence of the take-up of the care and facilities offered. A study is undertaken to show how many people were referred to the speech and language therapists with swallowing problems during the previous three years. Results would indicate whether the numbers of referrals had been rising, falling or staying the same during those years and could be used in estimates of staff time (man hours) being included in forward-planning.

In another setting, where a multidisciplinary approach to better integration of services is an immediate aim, management needs more information about the relative treatment input from three parallel departments – occupational therapy (OT), physiotherapy (PT) and speech and language therapy (SLT) – in two of its centres. Analysis of existing records covering a chosen period would allow comparison of caseloads and numbers of treatments for each of these departments. It would also show whether people had received well-planned programmes or had spent a lot of time keeping appointments that were not consecutive. An appropriate research question might compare the number and scheduling of treatments (OT, PT and SLT) given to stroke patients in the two centres under review.

3.5 CLINICAL TRIALS

As its name suggests, a **clinical** trial is carried out in a healthcare setting. Originally clinical trials were used to explore the response of human beings to a medication that had been developed and tested in the laboratories of the drug companies, basically to put a seal of safety and effectiveness on the new product. Their designs have been extended more recently to include investigations into advances in healthcare techniques and treatments in realistic situations.

A clinical trial has been described as:

> an experiment carried out to assess the effectiveness of a new treatment regime.
>
> Kirkwood (1988: 184)

The experimental design is intended to ensure that an experiment affords a valid, efficient and unambiguous test of the hypothesis set up and that extraneous variables are controlled.

Miller and Wilson (1983)

Design of clinical trials

Let us consider briefly the five most common variations in these trials.

- One group post-test
- One group pre-test–post-test
- Pre-test–post-test control group
- Post-test only control group
- Crossover design

One group post-test

Clinical trials of this type may be referred to as 'one shot case studies'. As the name implies, this design involves one group of subjects who all receive the treatment package and who are assessed after the course of treatment. In diagrammatic form, this can be shown as

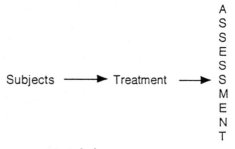

Figure 3.3 One-group post-test design.

However, there is an obvious problem in interpreting the results of such a study. There is no baseline with which to compare the final results. How would you know that subjects had a better score than they did before receiving the treatment package? The answer is simple: you would not know. Consequently such a trial design, although used in the past, is now considered inadequate.

One group pre-test–post-test

Again, as the name implies, there is one group of subjects who all receive the treatment package. In this design, however, tests are performed before the treatment begins and repeated afterwards. Thus there is a baseline measure of their performance. By comparing the two results you could find that the subjects' performance was:

- better
- worse
- unchanged.

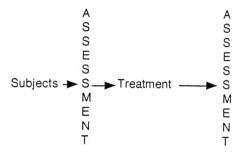

Figure 3.4 One-group pre-test post-test design.

So could we conclude that if the subjects gained better scores in the post-test that the treatment worked? The answer is 'No', and unfortunately a common error of interpretation made by some researchers would be to say 'Yes'. We could not make this conclusion because we would not know whether or not the people were improving independently of the treatment. In other words, they may have been improving naturally or because of some other factor. The improvement in their test performance would not necessarily be a result of the treatment we had given them. The only conclusion we could draw from such a trial would be that the observed improvement MIGHT HAVE BEEN DUE to the treatment.

Pre-test–post-test control group

In this design there are **two groups** of subjects who are both tested before and after the treatment period, although **only one group** receives the treatment. The second group acts as a control. What could we tell from the results this time?

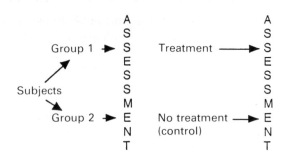

Figure 3.5 Pre-test post-test control group design.

- If group 1 shows more improvement than group 2 it could be concluded that the difference is due to the treatment: that is, the treatment is effective or working.

- If the improvement shown by the two groups is the same, it would seem that the treatment has no effect: that is, it does not work.

- If group 2 shows more improvement than group 1 it would suggest that not only was the treatment not working, it actually seems to be making people worse. (It would be wise to stop it immediately in case you are sued!)

This two group design therefore provides much more convincing evidence of the success or failure of the treatment being investigated.

Post-test only control group

This design is the same as the previous one apart from one factor: subjects are only assessed at the end of the procedure.

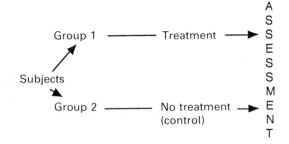

Figure 3.6 Post-test only control group design.

The argument for this design is that, provided the subjects are properly randomized (see section 2.3.1), there should be no difference in perform-ance between the groups before the treatment. This assumes that the baseline measurement would be the same for both groups and allows direct comparison of the post-test results, as in the previous design. The danger would be if one group, even with randomization, were to begin with an unknown and widely different performance from the other.

Crossover design

The general principles for crossover designs have been covered in section 2.3.2. In essence, whatever the experimental conditions, each of several groups is observed under all these conditions, but in a sequence that is not repeated for any other group. In a crossover clinical trial, all groups of subjects have the opportunity to receive the treatment at some time in the study.

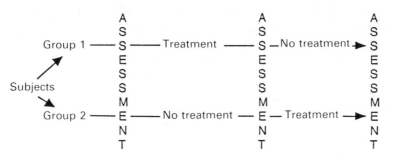

Figure 3.7 Crossover design.

For example, Burl, Williams and Nayak (1992) carried out a trial to explore the effect on walking balance of immobilizing the neck with a cervical collar. They recruited 20 subjects who were divided by age into two groups. All subjects were asked to wear flat shoes and not to drink any alcohol before the trial. To ensure that conditions would be the same, the under surface of the shoes being worn was cleaned before the test began. Each subject walked along the walkway twice, once while wearing a cervical collar and once without wearing the collar. To control for any practice or sequence effect, the authors randomized the 'collar' and 'no collar' conditions. The results did not demonstrate any differences between the two conditions and the authors were able to conclude that wearing a cervical collar had no effect on walking balance.

Randomized controlled trials

In some healthcare situations, the formal clinical trials we have discussed are not seen as fully appropriate. There is a strong opinion that it is not ethical to withhold treatment from patients while they are used as members of a control group. Yet it is generally agreed that new techniques should be evaluated in an objective way before they are adopted. Also, there are many treatments that have been in use for years without objectively assessing their effects: with growing numbers of people needing continuing care, we need to be sure of the value of any services we are providing. An applied version of the clinical trial, known as a RANDOMIZED CONTROLLED TRIAL (RCT), has a well-earned reputation for combining the rigour of a clinical trial with an acceptable interpretation of the pure 'no treatment' condition (Moffett, 1991).

Examples of RCTs

From the relatively small number of published RCTs within the para-medical professions, we have selected two examples:

Juby, Lincoln and Berman (in press, 1995) investigated the functional and psychological effects of different rehabilitation regimes for people who were recovering after a stroke. Patients were randomly allocated to either a stroke unit or to treatment on general medical or healthcare of the elderly wards. Those who received treatment in the stroke unit were seen to be more independent in daily living activities and were psychologically more able to cope with the changes in their ability than those who received rehabilitation on the conventional wards.

Drummond and Walker (1995) focused their study on leisure rehabilitation. Patients who had had a stroke were randomly allocated to one of three groups described as a leisure rehabilitation group, a conventional occupational therapy group and a control group respectively. Baseline assessments of leisure activities were carried out as each subject was recruited for the study. The assessment was repeated three months and six months after discharge from hospital. The results showed an increase in leisure scores for the leisure rehabilitation group but not for the other two groups. The authors concluded that providing a leisure rehabilitation programme for stroke patients does increase involvement in leisure activities.

Multicentre trials

Multicentre trials are valued in medical research, particularly because they provide a realistic way of recruiting large numbers of subjects in a reasonable time limit. Also, it is feasible to draw general conclusions from the results. Research therapists in rehabilitation centres are showing a growing interest in the advantages of this sort of collaboration.

3.6 SINGLE SUBJECT EXPERIMENTS/STUDIES

Over the years, scientists and thinkers have tried to find ways to account for the **variability** and **generality** of their observations. In spite of this, the true sources of variability have been very elusive, whether the researcher has focused on personal attributes (intrinsic factors of variability) or on conditions in the world around their subjects (extrinsic factors of variability). This has led scientists to assume that the greater part of variability is **random** in origin: if its sources cannot be found, individual variability should be discounted.

The best way to do this depends on making observations of large numbers of apparently similar people and then using statistical correction to eliminate the random variation. We have become used to research that has a carefully regulated design and can present results based on 'average' scores and 'normative' responses. Frequently, investigators generalize their findings from the group they have been observing to supposedly similar populations. Basically, the sources of individual variability have been calculated out of the situation. This characteristic is common to most of the methods discussed above in sections 3.1–3.4.

In contrast, single subject experiments and studies try to find out the sources of variability in an INDIVIDUAL. It could be argued that an obvious limitation of single case studies is that their findings cannot be generalized. However, not all researchers agree that this is the case:

> the more we learn about the effects of treatment on different individuals, in different settings, etc., the easier it will be to determine if that treatment will be effective with the next individual. If we ignore differences among individuals and simply average them into a group mean, it will be more difficult to estimate the effects on the next individual.
>
> Barlow and Hersen (1984)

An interesting paper by Wilson, Cranny and Andrews (1992) illustrates the potential of single case experimental designs. Using a series of pilot studies they investigated the effects of music on people in a prolonged coma. Their purpose was to find clear evidence, rather than anecdotes, to support the idea that comatose people can be aroused by their favourite music. In two of their studies there were:

> significant behaviour changes which suggested increased arousal, one showed decreased arousal after the stimulation period and one no change.
>
> Wilson, Cranny and Andrews (1992: 181)

Several approaches, relying on observation, are available for focusing on single subjects. These use **quantitative** and **qualitative** methods.

Quantitative studies in single subject studies

Quantitative studies involve repeated measurement of a single person over time, either maintaining the conditions of performance as constant as possible, for example, by checking the range of movement in a knee joint, following meniscectomy; recording the frequency or intensity of the problem behaviour of a patient within a series of art therapy sessions; or making periodic, reactive changes to environmental or treatment factors as these are judged necessary.

These two options have counterparts in the ways we organize treatment, on the one hand, for people who have a temporary problem and are expected to recover, and on the other for people who have a deteriorating disorder, with a poor prognosis. When repeated measurements are made in a health or social service setting, the subject profile usually shows whether the person has improved, stayed the same or become worse. The measurements may also show a pattern or cycle of improvement and deterioration which does not seem to be directly related to the treatment programme. In a single subject study, changing the treatment or the way the research design is applied, in response to any of these outcomes, can allow an immediate search for the SOURCES of variability in the subject.

Alternating treatment designs

The design details described for clinical trials (in section 3.5) can be applied to single case experiments. It is just as important to be precise in assessing your subject before and after any treatment, in order to have a baseline for comparison. The single subject acts as their own control and it is realistic to apply different treatment regimes (denoted as condition 'A' and condition 'B') in particular sequences, either to one person only or to a series of individual subjects, for example, ABA or BAB or ABBA, with an agreed period of rest between the three sets of conditions.

Qualitative studies in single subject studies

In these studies, the investigator actively seeks the reported experiences, opinions, attitudes and judgements of individual subjects. Semi-structured interviews and questionnaires that are used in such studies are characterized by open questions with freedom for the subject to spontaneously follow his reactions to topics that are introduced into the conversation or question- naire. If the study is based on grounded theory, work proceeds in stages. The wealth of anecdotal and freely expressed verbal material collected in the first stage is subsequently scanned for key words and common themes. These are 'fed into' the guidelines for semi-structured interviews and open questions for the next stage. This process continues until a core of constructs and ideas have crystallized from the data, enabling the investigator to generate theories that extend them. (For further information about grounded theory, see Chenitz and Swanson, 1986.)

Chapter 4 explores other research tools and functional tests that can be used with either single subjects or groups. It also considers the importance of standardized tests.

<table>
<tr><td>

4

</td><td>

Collection of data

</td></tr>
</table>

4.1 INTRODUCTION

Although the title for this chapter is straightforward enough it covers this and several related matters. The first section explores the principles of tests for assessing your subjects and assembling your observations. These are grouped under the heading of 'tools of enquiry' and range from standardized tests through checklists to health-related functional tests. This is followed by a discussion on the use of pilot studies which are used for checking all aspects of your research design for feasibility. I emphasize the importance of adjusting your questionnaire, or other measurement tool, if there are any difficulties with these. After pointing out some of the problems that can arise and giving some general advice, the chapter ends with a section on coding the data you have collected in preparation for their analysis.

4.2 TOOLS OF MEASUREMENT AND ENQUIRY

If you cannot measure it, you cannot manage it.

Old adage

The average length of researcher time required to develop a research tool to the point appropriate to use in a study is five years.

Reid and Boore (1987: 227)

You may feel that Reid and Boore give an unduly pessimistic view of the timescale for designing tests but, as we said earlier when discussing the construction of a questionnaire, there are no short cuts. Kerlinger (1986) sees test construction as a 'formidable job', although he acknowledges that because many performance tests were set up in educational settings, they cannot always be used in research which deals with health and social care.

If you have to design your own measurement tool, you will have to allow a realistic budget in time and money. But if there is an existing test that meets your research needs, it may be wise to use one that has already been thoroughly tested for its reliability and validity. Remember, it is possible for a test or procedure to be reliable (one for which test/retest scores are close or identical) but not valid, although it must be reliable if it is to be valid (it actually tests what it is said to test).

Standardized tests

Published tests come with precise instructions about the ways they may be used. These instructions include details of the space and equipment required, the time to be taken in completing the test and the exact wording to be used in explaining the responses you are asking your subjects to make. They have usually been standardized and they have tables of normative scores that are readily available.

> Standardised tests . . . are based on . . . content common to a large number of (educational) systems. They are the products of a high degree of professional competence and skill in test-writing and, as such, are usually quite reliable and generally valid.
>
> Kerlinger (1986: 451)

Bearing in mind the time that has to be invested in developing any research instrument, if there is a suitable test for the people you want to study, it leaves you more time to explore the questions you are asking in your project. However, it is never wise to alter a standardized test to 'fit' your target population by making serious changes in the original wording of the test items or by modifying the way it is used. Detailed advice on test construction can be found in Adkins (1974) or Edwards (1957).

Let us examine some of the topics and fields covered by standardized tests that might be used appropriately in your research. For the moment, these will not include the interview schedules and questionnaires discussed earlier in Chapter 3, but will focus on standardized tests and scales which have been developed within educational settings and in fields of behavioural and social sciences. Healthcare professionals may want to use them to check on the comparability of people, or groups of people, before beginning a study. Some of these tests have to be carried out by qualified psychologists but others are available for use by health professionals, particularly those who have attended a short course in test application. These courses are offered from time to time by the British Psychology Society (BPS) in collaboration with the National Federation of Educational Research (NFER). The professional associations are kept informed of the dates of courses: you may find you have colleagues in your department who have taken such a course or you may wish to contact either the BPS or NFER about future courses.

Tests make use of questions to sample knowledge or involve rating and ranking scales. They can be classified according to the focus of the test items as:

- achievement tests
- aptitude and intelligence tests
- attitude scales, value and interest scales
- personality measures.

You may decide that you need to check the similarities or differences between the people you are hoping to invite to take part in your project. It may be important for your study that you can refer to their attitudes, interests and personality if these are likely to influence your findings.

Achievement tests

These can be based on general or special areas of knowledge, exploring the person's understanding and also to what extent they have mastered and are proficient in using that knowledge. General knowledge achievement tests sample and measure the use of language, breadth of vocabulary, reading ability and basic skills in arithmetic. As a researcher, you may need to check whether your subjects have comparable levels of language and reading skills and whether these will allow them to understand what you will be asking them to do.

Aptitude and intelligence tests

Aptitude tests are often used in career counselling, for guiding people towards a range of suitable job choices. If we define aptitude as a capacity for learning and achievement, these tests could be used as an alternative to achievement tests in order to screen our possible subjects.

Intelligence tests are used regularly in educational settings and may also be used to evaluate the mental age of people with learning difficulties. In the latter situation, it is unusual for therapists to be involved formally in testing intelligence: it is more likely that the results of intelligence tests for any such client will be available in the client's notes.

A thorough review of intelligence tests, including 'omnibus' types that cover a wide range of skills, is available in Sax (1980) *Principles of Educational and Psychological Measurement and Evaluation*. There are also some published, standardized and well-known functional tests that therapists and other health professionals have prepared and validated for people with particular biopsychosocial needs. We will consider these separately.

Attitude scales, value and interest scales

Attitudes are said to reveal the organized beliefs and cognitive processes of perceiving, thinking and feeling which lead us to behave in an individual and consistent way towards the people, topics or objects around us. There is considerable overlap between attitudes, opinions and value judgements: it is even possible to consider that all these form part of a wider concept of personality. Generally, these factors have been explored by asking people to show the extent to which they agree or disagree with statements made on the test sheet. In other words, each subject is asked to rate their support for the statements. Often the statements are about sensitive topics such as human rights, religious freedom, social issues or political opinions.

There are three main styles of such **rating scales**. The first two are used more widely than the third. They are:

- summated rating scales, also known as **Likert-type** scales
- cumulative scales, also known as **Guttman** scales
- **equal-appearing interval** scales.

Likert scales

In Likert scales, all items are held to be of equal value in demonstrating attitude. The response choices have to be made from five or seven possibilities. These range from 'strongly agree', through 'undecided' to 'strongly disagree'. Results are obtained by adding the scores together and calculating their mean value. The results are open to bias which could be induced by people who are inclined to agree or disagree with *any* written statement or who tend to avoid making a decision (the 'don't know' syndrome).

A well-known example of a summated rating scale is the F-scale which measures authoritarian attitudes. The 'F' is derived from the parallel originally drawn between high authoritarianism and 'Fascism'. Although it has been challenged on the basis that it may not meet some criteria of validity, Kerlinger (1986) considers that it was well-constructed. The scale is based on more than 40 general statements which are combined in clusters. These clusters are linked to a range of traits that show authoritarian tendencies: people who agree with these statements score highly on authoritarianism. Statements 2, 26 and 34 (Adorno, 1950) are given as examples:

2. No weakness or difficulty can hold us back if we have enough will power.
26. People can be divided into two distinct classes: the weak and the strong.
34. Most of our social problems would be solved if we could somehow get rid of the immoral, crooked and feeble minded people.

Guttman scales

By contrast, a Guttman scale is designed with each successive item reflecting a rising intensity of attitude and aimed at measuring one variable only. The scale consists of small sets, say five, of similar but progressing items. These are organized so that if a person agrees with the first of the set, he will agree with the remaining four. The opposite is also true: if he responds negatively to the first item, it is extremely likely that the remaining items in the set will also have negative responses. Results are calculated from cumulative scores, with emphasis on the patterns of responses.

Equal-appearing interval scales

In making up an interval scale with equally weighted items, several statements are prepared to comment on the same behaviour, event or object. The views of teams of expert judges are collected about these statements before creating the actual scale. Each item is awarded a **scale value**, possibly 1–10 for a set of ten items, reflecting the level of agreement between judges. It is considered that there are equal intervals between the items of the scale and that the lowest scale value indicates the most POSITIVE attitude. For details about this form of attitude scale, see Thurstone and Chave (1929: 61–3).

Ranking tasks

Putting behaviour, events or objects into a RANK ORDER is an alternative to rating them. This method is often used in tests designed to measure interests and values alone, but it can also be used to good effect within a questionnaire. The subject is asked to allocate a RANK indicator (e.g. 1–5) to each of the items listed for consideration.

There are two ways in which RANKING may be used: these are known as normative and ipsative. In a normative ranking test, the subject can award any of the indicators (e.g. 1–5) as often as they wish. With an ipsative ranking task, each indicator can only be used once. From the point of view of the subject, the tasks are different but probably neither is more taxing than the other. However, many of the tests used in statistical analysis should not be used with results that depend on ipsative measures because the effects of 'chance' have been altered by limiting the use of the available ranks. It is wiser to use normative ranking tasks if you need them in a questionnaire.

Personality measures

Writings in applied psychology show some success in measuring personality, despite the major difficulty of identifying the concept so that the validity of proposed tests can be agreed. Most of the tests concentrate on particular

TRAITS that are held to be indicators of personality, while psychologists have proposed sharp distinctions between people on the basis of the way they behave. Although these distinctions have drawn attention to major differences in personality, such as those who are 'extroverts' and those who are 'introverts', observations show us that many people fit somewhere between the two in a category that might be called 'mixed'. Those who set up the description of contrasting personalities see them as being at either end of a continuum. A wide variation of personality traits can be accommodated on such a continuum.

In addition to their preference for cheerful, social interaction or quiet, solitary activities, people may have behaviours that show them to be 'arrogant', 'anxious', 'conscientious', 'considerate', 'domineering', 'humble', 'loyal', 'proud'. Personality tests have been developed to measure some of these dimensions. These tests either depend on items which, on the face of it, reflect the traits we observe or else they are designed to explore the theories about the relationship of any one trait to a range of other variables. These are said to have 'face validity' on the one hand and 'construct validity' on the other. Once again, as Kerlinger (1986) says, it is important to realize that test items may measure a tendency to agree with socially desirable statements rather than what we think they measure.

Observation tools

The standardized tests discussed above can be used to take baseline measures of the people who volunteer to be observed or interviewed in your study. When it comes to detailed planning of the interviews and observation sessions you need, it is essential that you design and keep to routines that can be repeated without variations. It is wise to have a written framework for all the actions to be taken. Individual researchers tend to develop their own ways of depicting and recording their work. Two possible aids to organization are the CHECKLIST and the INTERVIEW SCHEDULE.

Checklist

The construction of a checklist has some similarities with designing a questionnaire, as the observer is asked to make explicit choices from a displayed range of boxes or columns to be ticked or words to be circled. Observation is guided by a series of phrases which represent behaviours, communications, actions and/or interactions that have been selected for observation. The entries made by the observer show how often and at what intervals repeated behaviours occur or record the people who interact and the sort of communication(s) they use.

Exactly what is to be observed and how observations are to be recorded has to be decided in advance so that a suitable recording sheet can be prepared. This is usually done by listing the selected items on the left of the page with response spaces arranged to the right. It is important that any KEY or coding system is clear and understandable and that enough space is allowed for easy and quick recording. The best way to make sure that the checklist meets your requirements is to try it out in a pilot study and identify any necessary improvements or changes.

The final preparation of a checklist includes setting up a standard heading for the recording sheet. This usually has the title of the study and spaces for the date and time of the observation session, the name of the observer and a code for the subject or subjects being observed. If the research design includes a pre-test/post-test comparison, you may wish to print the two recording sheets on paper of different colours.

The sample checklist below was designed for observations on a group of four teenagers, with challenging behaviour, who have been referred for social skills training.

Interview schedule

In the case of interview schedules, the researcher prepares a framework to guide and support a series of interviews so that each one is conducted in the same way as all the others. A good schedule covers the time taken for each component of the interview as well as details of the wording and demonstrations to be used. For example, a structured interview usually has three parts: an introduction, a period of questioning and a conclusion. The detailed wording of the spoken part of the interview is likely to include:

Introduction

● welcoming the person to be interviewed and introducing yourself

● reaffirming that the subject is willing to be interviewed

● telling the subject that he/she is free to choose to end the session

● assuring the subject that anything said will be recorded anonymously and will be held in complete confidence

● explaining what is going to happen and giving guidance or instructions about anything that the subject is expected to do or say.

Questioning

● each question will be printed in full.

Conclusion

● inviting the subject's comments or questions

Community Mental Health Unit, Occupational Therapy Department

Group referral : Record of Observations

Aim .... *Social Skills Training*...Date...............................
Description of session *Question/answer in dyads + sharing equipment in 4s*
(preparation of Youth Club newsletter)

Name	Positive behaviours					Negative behaviours				
	partici-pates	asks qs pleasantly	answers qs pleasantly	shares equipmt.	smiles, nods	disrupts activity	asks qs rudely	does not answer	refuses to share equip	face angry, shakes head
Jim										
Mary										
Susan										
Tom										

KEY

Positive behaviours by columns

1. Participates appropriately in the activity.
2. Asks questions politely, initiates comments.
3. Answers questions politely, responds when spoken to.
4. Gives up equipment when asked.
5. Uses positive body language, smiles, nods head.

Negative behaviours by columns

1. Disrupts the group activity.
2. Asks questions aggressively, shouts.
3. Refuses to answer questions, will not continue conversation, is rude.
4. Refuses to share equipment when asked.
5. Uses negative body language, has angry expression, shakes head.

Instructions : without speaking, observe group for a 10 minute period ; enter a tick in the relevant column for each instance of behaviours in the key above against the name of the client. Repeat the observation, using a second blank form, after a 10 minute rest from observation. Sign both of the sheets you have completed.

Observer (block capitals)..

Signature ....

Figure 4.1 Sample checklist.

- closing the formal part of the interview with a standard sentence

- thanking the subject for cooperation and time given

- making sure that the subject has the appropriate means for the return journey.

Once again, a pilot study will either confirm the time estimates you have made for each part of the interview or show you where more (or less) time is required. It will also provide an opportunity to check that instructions and questions can be readily understood.

4.3 FUNCTIONAL AND HEALTH-RELATED PERFORMANCE TESTS

Working alone or with colleagues in parallel professions, therapists have developed special functional tests to measure the abilities and responses of their patients. These measures are used in initial assessments so that care and treatment goals can be agreed with the patient, family and carers. Subsequently, the measurement tools are used to chart progress and to show where procedures should be altered to reflect changing needs. Therapists need to know, on a frequent basis, how well their patients and clients can communicate, see, hear, control their movements, maintain posture and carry out everyday activities.

Many of the tests devised for answering questions about a person's independence and general functioning have been standardized for their target populations. Some of these have been through all the stages of formal publication, while others are available in professional journals or by direct request to the team who developed them. Tests that are available commercially are included in catalogues from several sources, particularly from the Psychological Corporation and NFER-Nelson (addresses are given at the end of this book in the section on further reading). Because revision and refinement of the tests is a continuous activity, it is best to buy the latest version of a test as close as possible to when you plan to use it, allowing time for postal delivery.

There is no point in trying to devise your own test unless this is absolutely necessary. Remember there is already a very large pool of tests available in books, journals and theses as well as those that are marketed commercially. As a rule of thumb, it is always preferable to choose well-established, recognized assessments. Read around your subject area (do a special literature search) and find out what other researchers have used. Good researchers will always highlight problems with particular tests in the discussion sections of their papers and this can provide invaluable help.

However, remember that there are always problems associated with the choice of test, even in well-known, well-used assessments. A few general points are worth bearing in mind:

1. Be clear about what you want to measure (IQ? Perception? Arm movement? Mood? Use of hospital services?). Ensure that you are as specific as possible. For instance, if you are researching the area of perception you may find a general perceptual assessment (such as the Rivermead Perceptual Assessment Battery, Whiting *et al.*, 1985) is appropriate. However, if you want to concentrate on a more defined area you may need to consider using another test, for example, Albert's Test of Neglect (Albert, 1973).
2. Be sure that the test is VALID.
3. Check for evidence of test RELIABILITY.
4. Consider the sample of subjects to be studied and decide if the test is suitable. For example, how long does the test take to administer? Would this be a reasonable time to expect the subject to spend within the test situation? Or, if the patient has aphasia, will this affect performance? Or, would a basic Activities of Daily Living (ADL) measure such as the Barthel Index (Mahoney and Barthel, 1965) be a suitable measure of ADL performance for a stroke patient two years after discharge from hospital?
5. Consider whether or not specific training is necessary in order to carry out the test. If it is not, decide whether the accompanying manual or guidelines are adequate. Look carefully at the scoring of the test. If you have any doubts, try out the test on some colleagues or patients who are willing to help.
6. Talk to others who are familiar with the test. Ask experts their opinion and sound out informed colleagues. Other researchers who are in the middle of a study often have florid views on assessments they are using.
7. Ask yourself 'Would another test be better?' No test is sacrosanct; each will have its limitations.

To illustrate these points more clearly, let us consider a well-known and well-respected assessment. The Barthel ADL Index, first developed by Mahoney and Barthel in 1965 and later modified by Collin *et al.* (1988) is used widely in the field of stroke research. Among its advantages are that:

- it has established evidence of validity
- it has good evidence of reliability
- it is simple to use and quick to score
- its wide usage means that results are easily communicable to other researchers and the findings of similar studies can be compared with yours.

However, it has been criticized because:

- it has a floor-and-ceiling effect in the scoring. The ceiling effect is an important consideration in rehabilitation research although it is usually overcome by using additional, extended ADL scales (for example, the Nottingham Extended ADL Scale, Nouri and Lincoln, 1987)
- therapists dislike the Barthel ADL Index because it is insensitive to small changes in performance. Nevertheless, it is as well to recognize that, in general, the more sensitive a scale is, the more unreliable it becomes
- subjects with the same score can have different abilities and therefore the index is an unsatisfactory way of comparing individuals
- there are some 'mutations' of the original Barthel ADL Index in existence. These cause some confusion about which measure has actually been used in a reported research project.

In summary, you have a very large array of possibilities when it comes to assessing your subjects. Choosing an appropriate test is a difficult task. READ around the field, TALK to colleagues and TRY OUT the test in question before you decide to adopt it for your study.

4.4 THE PILOT STUDY

This section looks at the process of fine-tuning the system you have planned for collecting information. Because most of the adjustments that your system needs will be in response to any ideas or problems uncovered by a pilot study, we deal with this first. Then we consider general strategies and precautions for data collection before exploring the coding process that enables you to prepare your data for analysis.

> expert advice and spurious orthodoxy are not substitutes for well-organised pilot work.
>
> Oppenheim (1966: 25)

The aim of the pilot study is to identify potential problems in the data collection and to show that the study design is both appropriate and feasible. It will also give some idea of the costs of the study as well as experience in carrying out the project. This is particularly useful if you are not completely familiar with the procedures or techniques involved. Treece and Treece (1977: 25) have defined the pilot study as 'a small preliminary investigation of the same general character as the major study, which is designed to acquaint the researcher with problems that can be corrected in preparation for the large research project'. It may be more simply defined as a small-scale trial of the research you are undertaking.

Many researchers mistakenly view a pilot study as extra work or just a time-wasting exercise. If the pilot study is a complete success you may feel justified in feeling this way. However, more commonly, you will come across problems that will make you glad that you invested the time and trouble in piloting your study.

Pilot interviews are particularly important because they allow potential interviewers the opportunity to practise being consistent and to practise reflection and prompting skills if the research calls for them. It is vital that where there are obvious discrepancies between several interviewers, these are resolved by, for example, providing guidelines to make sure that everyone does the same. Thus any problems identified can be ironed-out in the preliminary stages before going on to the actual study.

The group of subjects used for the pilot study must be as similar as possible to the group you wish to study. Although valuable information can be obtained by circulating the draft form of a questionnaire to your colleagues, this will not be as illuminating as sending it to subjects who are similar to your study population. Subjects who will be taking part in the main project should not be involved in the pilot study: it could be argued that they would modify their answers with practice and would have an advantage over other subjects who have no previous knowledge of the questionnaire.

Bearing in mind that many potential problems can be uncovered, we now consider some examples obtained from piloting a questionnaire. The list is by no means exhaustive.

Some questions are not answered

This may be because subjects do not understand the question, they do not know the answer to the question or they do not have time to complete the answer.

Subjects misunderstand a question because it is ambiguous

Example 1 'Are stairs a problem for you?' Potentially this could be seen as a request for information about mobility problems, preference for ground-floor accommodation, decorating problems or general difficulties associated with stairs as opposed to specific problems with using stairs at home. To make sure the subject gives the answer that is needed, the question should ask: 'Do you have any difficulty in climbing up your stairs at home?'

Example 2 'Is dressing a problem?' This question could be asking for information on a wide range of topics: physical problems in getting dressed, the amount of time involved in dressing, difficulties in finding fashionable clothes or the actual expense of buying new clothes. In this case, the researcher meant to ask 'What physical problems do you have in dressing yourself?'

All subjects record the same response to a question, so it has no value as a discriminator

In a study exploring the quality of life for people with haemophilia, for example, it would be a waste of time to record if subjects were MALE or FEMALE since the disease only occurs in males.

The questionnaire takes much longer to complete by subjects than was anticipated

This may mean that the last questions are not completed or that the answers are rushed and lack detail. Such a questionnaire should be reviewed and reduced; the most important questions should occur as early as possible.

The costs are much higher than anticipated

You need to consider cheaper quality paper, giving questionnaires directly to people attending Out-patients rather than posting them, streamlining visits so that you visit geographical areas to reduce travel costs or, indeed, excluding subjects who live outside a specified catchment area.

Other factors that affect the study

This could be anything:

- other staff who do not understand the study giving incorrect information

- problems in identifying and recruiting subjects

- administrative difficulties, such as the forms are not easy to complete by subjects and researchers or there is not enough space left to record responses

- other practical problems: the equipment breaks down, is inappropriate, does not record correctly or is not available when it is needed, or there is difficulty in interviewing subjects on the ward because of noise, visiting times, time needs of other professionals on the patients.

All such headaches need to be sorted out before the major study begins.
    Pilot studies can, however, fail to highlight all flaws. This may be due to limiting factors such as time constraints, using an unrepresentative sample or, most commonly, not using enough subjects. How large should a sample

for the pilot study be? The figure advised is usually an arbitrary one, the chief ingredient in selecting the figure being common sense. If you expect to involve 1000 people as subjects in your project, it is useless to carry out a pilot using ten subjects. Similarly, if you mean to use 20 subjects, 15 subjects for the pilot study may be considered excessive. Treece and Treece (1977) suggest a guideline of 10% of the intended study sample and personally I feel this is reasonable.

Even if you decide that your actual study is going to be too small to merit running a pilot study, remember it is better to pilot your research tool on colleagues than on nobody at all. However, it is equally important to remember that there is a difference between professional colleagues who are familiar with medical terms and the people who will actually answer the questions in your major study. The pilot study alone will not identify all the flaws in a potential study. It is the COMBINATION of the pilot study with a sound knowledge of the relevant literature and discussion with experienced colleagues that will eliminate the obvious problems. The combination of factors is depicted in Figure 4.2. The best advice is to avoid looking at these areas in isolation from one another.

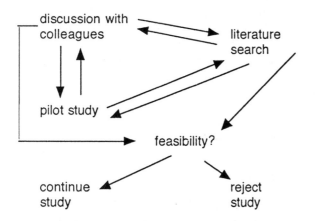

Figure 4.2 Judging the merits of a research proposal design.

One final word of warning: be careful of contamination when conducting a pilot study. You need to be careful that the pilot study does not alter the situation you are attempting to assess. For example, suppose you want to study the effect of certain exercises on recovery pattern. You may pilot this programme with several patients on a ward to see if they understand the instructions and can actually perform the movements. However, you may find that these subjects tell other patients about the exercises, other patients on the ward see and copy the programme or nursing and therapy staff implement the regime. In each of these instances the result is that the other patients begin to do the exercises you are evaluating and therefore cannot be used as controls. Do not underestimate the effect on your project of other staff teaching the exercises or using the activities they have seen you using during the pilot study. This may affect the overall regime on the ward thereafter, so you would never be able to recruit controls from this ward.

It is important to pilot ALL parts of the research process in order to identify any flaws in the design. Many students only pilot the collection of data, but you also need to pilot analysing the data and the ways of presenting your findings. Thus in addition to uncovering problems with data collection, you can identify potential pitfalls in the choice of statistical test and in choosing the most appropriate information to present. You may also discover that you are collecting too much material. Evans (1978: 61) advised 'Get all the information you need and no more.'

Problems identified in the pilot study must be set right before moving on. Ideally if there are major changes made to the study you should carry out a further pilot study using the amended design and research tools. Although this is advisable, time and money constraints may not allow you to do more than one pilot study. In this case, the best policy is to be as thorough as possible in revising the wording of the questionnaire, reducing its length if necessary and checking the venue and timing of interviews. When you are satisfied with the results of the pilot study, you can start on data collection for the major study.

It is wise to make a full record of what you did both in testing your design and questionnaires and in responding to the findings of the pilot study, although some researchers prefer to wait until they have finished their entire project before writing up this important stage of the whole process. However, information recorded formally about your pilot study can be valuable as a teaching aid and can also generate interest in a new area or approach.

For example, Sylvester (1990) conducted a pilot study comparing two treatments of patients who had osteoarthrosis (OA) of the hips. Fourteen patients were allocated to two groups to compare the effects of hydrotherapy with those of a combination of shortwave diathermy and exercise. There were significant differences between the groups with regard to pain, function and life satisfaction before and after treatment. Subjects receiving hydrotherapy had greater function and higher life-satisfaction scores. These results suggest that a larger study could indicate the benefits of hydrotherapy over other treatments with this patient group.

In a further example, McGuire and Greenwood (1990) carried out a pilot study on 18 patients with traumatic head injury. The researchers studied the effects of a memory programme on the patients' self-esteem and found that this improved. They concluded that more research in this area was needed using a larger number of patients and a control group.

4.5 GENERAL STRATEGIES

Organization is the key to efficient and effective data collection. You must allow time in your timetable:

1. For the data to be collected. This includes time for interviewing and/or treating subjects and travelling between subjects and centres. Where applicable, time must also be allowed for checking hospital records and admission lists.
2. For writing up notes. This must be done on a regular basis. Notes should be legible with no shorthand or personal abbreviations (they may not make sense several months later). Each assessment and piece of paper should have the subjects' surname/number and be dated.

   Record any special problems which may affect your results. For example, in a study of the treatment of hemianopia, make notes on subjects who have cataracts or who normally wear glasses. You WILL NOT remember this information at a later date.

   Time must also be made available for coding data where this is relevant.
3. For regular contact with your supervisor or mentor, if applicable.
4. For administration. Time is needed for organizing appointments, making telephone calls and liaison with other colleagues, particularly those involved in your research.
5. For self-development. Other research commitments, such as attending meetings and journal clubs, are important. Allow time for chasing up references, ordering journals and articles, reading papers, learning to use a computer: whatever is applicable to the success of your study.

Also ensure that you:

- make a copy of important data at regular intervals. These copies should be stored separately from the master copy

- are not tempted to check or analyse results halfway through a trial 'just to see how its going'. You may introduce bias which may subsequently mask important information

- have a telephone number where subjects or staff can leave messages or consult you about queries arising from the study

- carry a notebook for recording important information. Do not get into the habit of writing on scraps of paper which are alway misplaced

- record appointments in a diary and learn to consult this every time you arrange to see someone in connection with your study.

Finally, conduct the study honestly. Be as objective as possible and record information as you find it. Calnan (1976: 110) underlined the importance of this when he noted: 'This is the one fundamental demand in research, to be honest at all costs.'

4.6 POTENTIAL PROBLEMS

Hockey (1985: 29) had the following warning for researchers who believed that their research was so well-planned that nothing could go wrong:

> Let me tell you, it can, it usually does and it helps to know that it happens quite often.

Common problems that researchers complain of include:

Initially you have too much free time
Use this time wisely. You will regret it later if you do not. Prepare questionnaires, photocopy relevant information, read articles, draft instructions for others, check that any equipment works, that it records accurately and that you know how to use it.

The phenomenon of the disappearing subject
Anyone who has had any connections with research will tell you about the phenomenon of the disappearing subject. Even if you are studying one of the commonest disorders known to Man, you can guarantee that the incidence will drop during the study period. This phenomenon is known among the research fraternity as MURPHY'S LAW which says that no matter how much preparation you have made, and regardless of how many patients there were with the diagnosis or problem of interest before the research project, every potential subject will vanish when recruitment begins. Another important 'law' is O'REILLY'S LAW which simply states that Murphy's Law is optimistic. Sadly when this happens all you can do is wait.

Subjects withdraw
For a wide variety of reasons subjects may withdraw or become excluded from your research (see section 1.3 on ethical considerations). There is nothing you can do when people say they do not want to continue except to be polite to them, even if you scream in private.

Changes in staff occur
People associated with your research become ill, get pregnant or leave.

Again, be polite and understanding and clench your fists under the table.

Opinions change
Where your research was once welcomed gratefully, you have a feeling that staff groan when they see you coming. Ensure that you do not cause unnecessary inconvenience to others, be appreciative of the help you are given and keep others as up-to-date on your study as possible.

Variables change
Someone else changes an aspect of the subjects' management or environment. This can range from changing methods of admissions to a ward to changing a treatment regime or some other aspect of care. Whatever the change, the variables in the trial have been altered. Such an alteration in circumstances needs discussion with your mentor or other research colleagues. Do not just ignore the changes and hope for the best. Make a full record of any corrective decisions you reach and of the expected consequences for your project.

Transport problems
Your car breaks down or your subjects' transport breaks down, fails to collect them or is late. Remember to build extra time into your programme to allow for the unexpected.

Finance
Costs increase and the amount of finance allocated to the research is no longer adequate. Is it possible to apply for more money or to reduce costs in any way? Write down carefully all expenses involved so that you can get an overall idea of what is the biggest drain on resources. Ask the finance officer for advice.

Other
This can range from the photocopier breaking down through national strikes (ancillary, postal, power, transport) to an unexpected change in the weather. All these seemingly remote factors will affect your research. It is important to allow some leeway in your time estimates so that the whole study will not collapse if you are a few days out from your original plans.

4.7 CODING DATA

According to Bryman (1989: 49), the process and purpose of coding the raw information from a survey or experiment is 'the assignment of numbers to each answer category so that common answers can be aggregated.'

Regardless of the type of study you have decided to carry out, you will find that it is impossible just to analyse the data exactly as you have collected it. Many researchers prefer to begin coding their data as soon as they start collecting it instead of leaving it all to the end of their study.

To make it possible to manage a variety of different data, it must be represented by symbols or codes that indicate categories of information. The categories you use have to be arranged so that they are

1. *Mutually exclusive*
   This means that each datum can only fit into ONE of the available categories. Figure 4.3 shows a set of categories that fail to meet this standard because the limits of the categories overlap. Because these categories are not mutually exclusive, how would you know which category to use for someone who is 30 years old or someone who is 45 years old?
2. *Exhaustive*
   ALL possible answers and responses can be fitted into one of the available categories. Referring to Figure 4.3 again, we see that the set of categories extends from 18 to under 61 (61<). Because these age categories are not exhaustive, how could you allocate a subject who is 17-years-old?

   In contrast, Figure 4.4 illustrates a set of categories that is both mutually exclusive and exhaustive.

The coding system must be as simple as possible and, where more than one researcher is involved, there must be agreement between them about the coding of the information (inter-rater agreement). The reason for this is

Age categories for sample

Category	1	18–30
	2	30–45
	3	45–60
	4	61<

Figure 4.3 Example of overlapping categories.

Age categories for sample

Category	1	18 and under (<18)
	2	19–30
	3	31–45
	4	46–60
	5	61 and over (61<)

Figure 4.4 Example of mutually exclusive and exhaustive age categories.

obvious. If researchers coded the same information in different ways, it could affect the results of a research project. For example, if subjects with the same dressing ability were rated as '3' by one therapist and as '4' by another before commencing different treatments, how would the researcher be able to tell thereafter who had improved, who had not changed or who had deteriorated?

Coding closed questions

Data generated from closed questions (see section 3.3) are relatively easy to code. Essentially what you are doing is translating words into numbers so that your computer can make statistical sense of the information. For example, the computer will not understand the terms 'male' or 'female', but if you allocate each of these categories a code the computer can process the information. This could be: Male 0; Female 1. A code can also be developed to represent missing data for all the categories, providing this number will not be used elsewhere (e.g. Missing data 9).

If the first step is developing the code, the second is doing the actual coding. You may chose either to use the actual interview schedule or questionnaire. Many researchers use a 'FOR OFFICE USE ONLY' column on their forms and code here, see Figure 4.5.

		Office use
Q2 Are you . . .	Single	0
	Separated	1
	Divorced	2
	Widowed X	③
	Married	4

Figure 4.5 Example of a coding system.

Other researchers develop a coding sheet for each subject involved, see Table 4.1. These data-coding sheets have the advantage that they can be entered onto the computer relatively quickly and avoid the problems of fumbling over several pages of questionnaire.

Coding open questions

These are much more difficult to code as the subject is not limited in their choice of response (see section 3.3). Breakwell (1990: 86) astutely noted:

There will be problems in determining what categories to use in the content analysis. You are essentially taking a knife and chopping

Table 4.1 Example of an individual coding sheet

Name of subject . . . . Date . . . .

NOTE: **Range** of codes are given in brackets per question.

Where a response does not fit into the available codes, use **OTHER = 9**

		Code number	Comments
Closed questions			
group (treated/control)	(1, 2)		
age	(1–5)		
gender	(0 or 1)		
marital status	(1–4)		
diagnosis	(1, 2)		
Question 1	(1–5)		
Question 2	(1–3)		
Question 3	(1, 2)		
Question 4	(1, 2)		
Question 5	(1, 2)		
Open questions Question 6 (1–8 by key words)			
Question 7 (1–8 by key words)			
Question 8 (1–8 by key words)			
Question 9 (1–8 by key words)			
Question 10 (1–8 by key words)			

information into chunks. You may have difficulty knowing where to slice.

There are two main ways used to code open responses. You either have a predetermined list of expected replies and code the data accordingly. For example, the responses to the question 'What were your feelings about receiving treatment at home?' could be categorized under positive and negative replies. Or you can wait and see what the subjects actually say in reply to the various questions and then make appropriate codes.

In reality it is often difficult to find appropriate categories that adequately cover responses and it is sometimes necessary to use more than one category.

Coding error

Human error is likely to happen at some point in the coding process, either in allocating an actual category number, in transcribing the allocated code number or in entering it into the computer. However, as such errors are essentially random in nature, they are not likely to cause serious bias (Weisberg and Bowen, 1977: 73).

Helpful tips

1. Make sure that the subjects' number is on every piece of paper that relates to them.
2. Code information in large batches. In this way you memorize the codes and can use them more quickly and efficiently. Also, if there is a lot of information to code, you are less likely to try to interpret it as you go along, so there is less chance of you influencing the results by developing and introducing bias.
3. Enter the coded data into the computer in large sets. This is for the same reasons that I advise carrying out the coding in large batches.
4. Do not code and use a computer programme at the same time. If you keep the activities separate you will be more likely to detect unusual (potentially wrong) data.
5. Make printouts of entered data at regular intervals. Check that the information in these hard copies is correct and in the right columns. Always keep copies of these interim printouts, together with a record of any adjustments or corrections you have made on the computer spreadsheet.

5 | Analysis and presentation of data

A research study is no better than the quality of the analysis.
                                        Treece and Treece (1977: 265)

This section of the book deals specifically with the analysis of data. However, if you leave consideration of how to analyse your data until after it has been collected, you will almost certainly be in serious trouble. Consideration of the method of data analysis must be carried out as part of the planning process before the study actually begins. It is important to seek the help of an expert as early as possible in order to avoid obvious mistakes. Just as you would call in a plumber to cope with a problem in your plumbing or the gas board to sort out a gas leak, you need an expert to advise you on your analysis, particularly when statistics are involved. Hockey (1985: 27) puts this concisely:

> Enlist the help of a statistician at the very beginning of your work, even before the pilot study and try to find someone who does not mind helping the most pitiful ignoramus.

Her words reflect some of the nervousness that a first-time researcher may bring to the whole question of coming face to face with yet another unknown field. There is a pressing need to become familiar at least with the purposes and potential of statistics, but it is encouraging to read that everyone setting out on a research project looks for an ally in the statistical camp.

The analysis of the data you collect should not be seen as a minor part of your research study; it is one of the most important aspects to be considered. Lincoln (1990) rightly commented:

many studies contribute less than they might due to inadequacies in the methods of analysis.

While you are not expected to become a skilled analyst overnight, you will find it helpful to explore the principles on which measurement and analysis depend. This chapter deals first with the levels and uses of measurement and then with the general characteristics of statistics before touching on other forms of analysis and finishing with the ultimate purpose of the whole exercise: drawing conclusions from the outcome of your analysis. The subsections of the chapter are:

5.1 Levels of measurement
5.2 Statistics: a general introduction
5.3 Descriptive statistics
5.4 Inferential statistics
5.5 Use of a computer
5.6 Drawing conclusions

5.1 LEVELS OF MEASUREMENT

There is a convention for classifying measurements and placing them in one of four levels of precision. These are called nominal, ordinal, interval and ratio scales of measurement. For practical purposes, interval and ratio scales are often considered together. From the lowest to the highest level, the scales have different characteristics that determine and limit how you can apply arithmetical and statistical processes to them.

5.1.1 Nominal scale

This is considered to be the lowest and simplest level of measurement. Nominal measures are used to classify or label (i.e. give a name to) people, creatures, objects, behaviours or events. Any of these can be assigned to categories that must be: a) mutually exclusive – the limits of each category are separate from those on either side of it, so that an observation can be **'fitted into' only one** of them; b) exhaustive – there are sufficient categories to allow every observation to be assigned, **no observation has to be 'left out'** of the process of categorization. To make sure that all possibilities have been covered, it is usual to provide an ultimate category nominated as 'other'.

Examples of nominal categories:

- male/female
- dead/alive

- single/married/divorced/separated/widowed

- English/Irish/Scottish/Welsh/other.

Although nominal data indicate **differences**, they do not attribute any **value** to these categories. For example, in a questionnaire survey, we asked a group of subjects: 'Do you take exercise?'

Apart from providing information on the actual number of subjects who fall into each subgroup, no other facts are available from their answers to this question. For those who replied that they do take exercise, we do not know the amount of exercise taken, when or how often it is taken or the reason it is taken. Similarly, there is no information available about the reasons for not taking exercise from the other subgroup, nor do we know if they spend their time on other activities instead.

5.1.2   Ordinal scale

According to Wright and Fowler (1986), ordinal scales 'represent the most primitive level of numerical measurement'. This scale indicates a rank order in which things are arranged from the greatest to the least, the best to the worst. In such a scale, 3 is greater, or better, than 1, but it is impossible to claim that the difference between 3 and 1 is the same as the difference between 3 and 5. So it is easy to tell the **order** of the observations in relation to one another but no information is available on actual values.

For example, if you were given an ordinal scale of the weights of a group of people, you could tell the heaviest from the lightest but you would have no idea of the actual weight of each person.

Other examples: people could be placed in rank order on the basis of attributes such as:

- height: arranged from tallest to shortest

- examination results: arranged from best to worst

- staff seniority: arranged from consultant to junior doctor

- function: arranged from independent to dependent.

Once information has been placed in rank order it can be coded for processing by giving a number (1–X) to each rank. Referring to the example of ranking by height, in a group of 25 people, the tallest would be given the rank of 1 while the shortest would have the rank of 25. If two people were exactly the same height, both being equally deserving of the **fourth** place, they would be said to have 'tied' for the rank in question and a calculation would be needed to settle this fairly. We would have to award the rank of 4.5 to both of them, and use rank 6 for the person coming next in the list. In other words, the system combines the ranks that these people are competing for $(4 + 5 = 9)$ and divides it by the **number of potential candidates**, in this case, two. Where more than two people are candidates for the same rank, a similar calculation is necessary, adding the rank numbers that are open to competition and dividing the sum by the number of candidates for the highest of these ranks. This would result in a figure that could then be allocated to each candidate before returning to the original rank numbers once the 'tied' ranks have been settled.

5.1.3 Interval and ratio scales

These scales are at the most sophisticated and most precise levels of measurement. Numerical values are assigned to each observation or measurement taken.

Interval scales

These are usually shown as beginning with a zero point but there can be no real zero or absolute value for it. For example, the reading of 0° in temperature does not have any real meaning because it is impossible to envisage a situation with no temperature. Similarly it is impossible to say that a student therapist who obtains zero in an examination has absolutely no knowledge of the subject being examined. With interval scales it is also impossible to make judgements about any measurement in terms of any other or related value. We cannot say that a room with a temperature of 60° is TWICE AS WARM AS a room with a temperature of 30°. All that we can say is that the interval between 0° and 30° is the same as that between 30° and 60°. This is because there is no absolute zero point. The units of the scale are determined arbitrarily and we only know with confidence that there is an equal distance between the units.

Ratio scales

By comparison with interval scales, the ratio scale does have an absolute zero point which has a real meaning and therefore it offers an absolute measure. For example, it is possible to have no shoulder flexion, no blood pressure and no pulse. A ratio scale therefore provides the most precise information of all the measurement scales.

Although we have considered them separately and shown that there are some differences between interval and ratio scales, from the point of view of calculations within statistical analysis they can be managed as one category. Depending on how it has been collected, it is possible to have information that fits into any of the categories discussed. Blood pressure (BP), for example, can be expressed and recorded either as a ratio – 120/90 mmHg – or using an ordinal scale and referring to high/normal/low BP.

5.2 STATISTICS: A GENERAL INTRODUCTION

There are three kinds of lies, lies, damned lies and statistics.

Disraeli

Statistics are like a bikini! What they reveal is interesting. What they conceal is vital.

Robinson (1977: 160)

What are statistics?

Statistics have been defined as 'the science of collecting, summarising, presenting and interpreting data, and of using them to test hypotheses' (Kirkwood, 1988: 1). Statistics are important in research because they provide a vehicle for summarizing, understanding and communicating the information revealed by an investigation. However, it would be wise to remember the advice of Rowntree (1981) 'as a consumer of statistics, act with caution: as a producer, act with integrity'. Statistics are useful in making sense of the information we have collected but, to put it bluntly, they can be used fraudulently to make information appear better or worse than it actually is. Huff (1954) has written an excellent book on this subject. He provides examples from all areas of life, including newspapers, magazines and advertising. He has coined the term STATISTICULATION which he defines as 'misinforming people by the use of statistical material' (96).

Appropriately used, statistics enable us to present our data clearly. They help us to condense and make a comprehensive summary of what we have found out. Where relevant, statistics make it possible to accept or reject the null hypothesis of our study. To explore them further, we consider them under two headings: descriptive statistics and inferential statistics.

5.3 DESCRIPTIVE STATISTICS

Descriptive statistics can be used to prepare understandable explanations of your data in an economical way. Raw data are not interesting because they are meaningless. Number 'crunching' is essential in order to present information in an orderly fashion and to describe the most interesting characteristics of the data you have accumulated. The term 'descriptive statistics' is used to cover both GRAPHIC STATISTICS and SUMMARY STATISTICS.

5.3.1 Graphic statistics

These are characterized by drawings such as simple diagrams which can convey much more than paragraphs of words or long lists of numbers. The key to their effect is 'simple': a few simple diagrams or tables are more successful than those that are complicated or overloaded with information. Unless you want to provide a direct comparison of sets of information, it is a good idea to vary the type of display you see. Rows of pie charts may be boring to the reader because of their similarity and consequently some valuable information they contain may be missed. It is usually best to use a mixture of illustrations. There should never be any doubt why a diagram or table has been included in a presentation. They should never be used as 'padding'. They should illuminate the results and it must therefore always be clear what they relate to. The most commonly used graphic statistics are:

- Tables

- Graphs; histogram, bar graph, frequency polygon

- Pie charts

- Pictograms.

Tables

A table should be self-explanatory and able to stand alone. So it must have:

- a clear, informative title

- no abbreviations unless they are covered by an explanatory 'key'

- total values (e.g. n = 30, meaning that there were 30 subjects in all).

The most common mistake in tabular diagrams is to present an excessive amount of information. A good table is clear, easy to read and not overloaded with data. One variable can be compared with another by using CROSS-TABULATION: that is, plotting two sets of information on the same table. This is a good way to demonstrate a relationship, for example, by putting the age of clients and the amount of equipment supplied to them in one table.

The first step in summarizing data is often to construct a FREQUENCY DISTRIBUTION. To do this, a list of the categories involved is made and the number of times each variable occurs is counted. Each count is known as a 'frequency'. Suppose that we wanted to know the marital status of patients admitted for a total hip replacement (THR) in January, since their discharge plans might depend on their home and family environment. We could construct a frequency distribution table, summarizing the pertinent facts.

Table 5.1 Marital status of patients admitted to Fleming ward for THR, Jan. 19XX

Marital status	No. of occurrences	Frequency
Single	ЖГ ЖГ I	11
Married	ЖГ ЖГ ЖГ ЖГ ЖГ	25
Divorced	ЖГ I	6
Separated	III	3
Widowed	ЖГ ЖГ	10
Total		55

The frequencies may also be presented as **percentages** which would then be known as RELATIVE FREQUENCIES. For the example above, the relative frequencies would be 20%, 45.5%, 11%, 5.5% and 18% respectively. These can be entered and displayed as:

Figure 5.2 Marital status of patients admitted to Fleming ward for THR, Jan. 19XX

Marital status	Frequency	Relative frequency %
Single	11	20
Married	25	45.5
Divorced	6	11
Separated	3	5.5
Widowed	10	18
Total	55	100

It would also be possible to display these data in a graph or a pie chart. The sections below explore these options and offer guidelines for their use.

Graphs

The term 'graph' may be used to refer to histograms, bar graphs or frequency polygons. Each of these can be used to illustrate a frequency distribution in a clear, eye-catching way. Briefly, the values of the variable being studied are entered along the horizontal axis (the x axis) while the possible frequencies are entered in ascending order on the vertical axis (the y axis). You can check on this rule in the graphs shown below.

Histogram

The display given by a histogram reflects the continuous nature of the variable being depicted. Because of this, there are no spaces between the limits of the categories shown at the base of each histogram, that is along the horizontal axis. Using the data collected about people admitted for THR in January 19XX:

Marital status of patients admitted to Fleming ward for THR, Jan. 19XX

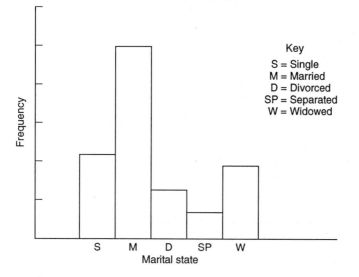

Figure 5.1 Example of a histogram.

The histogram is sometimes confused with the bar graph. The difference between these two forms of display is that there are spaces between the bars representing the frequencies of a bar graph while those of a histogram are touching each other. In other words, when you look at a bar graph, you are not meant to infer that the categories on the x axis (horizontal axis) are continuous.

Bar graph
The bars in a bar graph can be presented vertically or horizontally but all of them must be the same width and their height should indicate the magnitude of the observed frequency. Each part of the graph has to be clearly labelled and it is possible to enter figures/values inside the bars. The bar graph below illustrates one aspect of a study which investigated service to people with rheumatoid arthritis. It shows the number of patients who were supplied with tap turners during each month of 19XX (see Fig. 5.2)

A **composite bar graph** can be used to illustrate subdivisions of the general data. It is wise to observe some basic rules in constructing this type of chart:

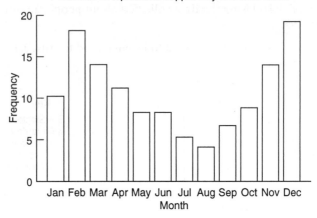

Figure 5.2 Example of a bar graph.

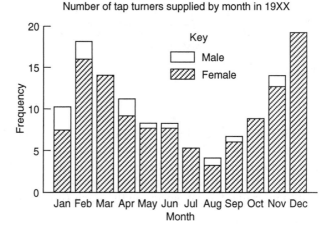

Figure 5.3 Example of a composite bar graph.

- set yourself a maximum of four components to include in each bar
- put the subdivision with the greatest frequency overall at the base of each bar
- use the same order for the subdivisions in each bar
- when you use shading to show the subdivisions, keep the darkest for the most important one.

If the data in our first illustration of a bar graph is now considered in terms of the gender of the people who received the tap turners, we can construct a composite bar graph. The bars will have the same height as before but they will be shaded to show how many women and how many men were given this equipment each month. Notice that a Key is used to indicate which shading applies to women and which to men (see Fig. 5.3).

Frequency polygons
Any data that can be presented in a histogram may be plotted as a frequency polygon. Basically, a cross is plotted at the midpoint of the top line of each column in the histogram. In height, this will coincide with the frequency the column represents. These points are then joined. The resulting line can be left 'floating' or it may be carried on as a dotted line until it intersects with the axis. The dotted line indicates that it does not represent any additional data. Using our data about tap turners again, they can be displayed in the form of a frequency polygon as shown below.

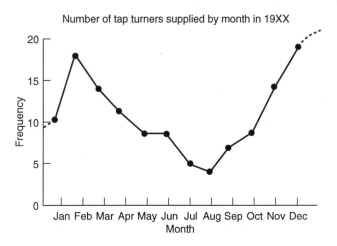

Figure 5.4 Example of a frequency polygon.

Pie charts

A pie chart is based on a circle which represents the total amount of information available for display. As its name suggests, the circle, or 'pie', is divided into segments so that the area of each segment is proportional to the number of observations it depicts. This sort of chart is a suitable choice for showing the proportions of classes of information to each other and to the data as a whole. To construct an accurate pie chart, two calculations are necessary. First, the frequencies or scores have to be converted into percentages. Second, these percentages have to be worked out in terms of their values in degrees, since there are 360 degrees available in a full circle.

For example, in a questionnaire, 20 out of 60 therapists indicated they might need to take maternity leave in the next two years. To represent this finding in a pie chart we would

- convert the raw number to a percentage: $20/60 \times 100 = 33.33\%$
- convert the percentage to degrees.

There are two arithmetical routes to the result needed:

either   60 therapists   (100%)   = 360 degrees
          20 therapists   (33.33%)   = 33.33 divided by 100 × 360
                                         = 119.99, rounded to 120 degrees

or   60 therapists   (100%)   = 360 degrees
           1 therapist   (1%)   = 360/60 = 6 degrees
          20 therapists   = 6 × 20 = 120 degrees

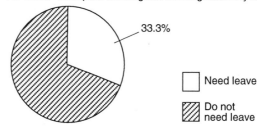

Pie chart: Therapists needing/not needing maternity leave

Figure 5.5 Example of a pie chart.

The pie chart can then be prepared, using a protractor, and labelled to indicate those therapists who might require maternity leave in the next two years as a proportion of those who responded.

If several pie charts are to be used when you are comparing data, each of them must have the same radius so that direct and accurate visual comparisons can be made.

Probably because of their relative ease of construction, there is a current tendency for pie charts to be overused. Remember that your readers need a variety of displays to hold their interest and to increase the chances that they pay attention to all the information you need to pass on. You will find a good example of the use of pie charts and other ways of displaying results in an article by Sutcliffe (1992).

Pictograms

Pictograms are made up from pictures or symbols which are used to represent data. They usually share some of the visual characteristics of the people or things that have featured in the pool of information, so they convey information very quickly. They might look like people if the project had been investigating staff numbers or family size, whereas they might look like houses if the study had focused on the rate of housing development in a suburban area. However, they are not good for accurate presentations, particularly when fractions are involved. They also tend to be used more commonly in advertising as they are more difficult to draw than graphs and their production can be costly.

There are two main types of pictograms:

1. Each symbol represents a specific value. An example of this type of pictogram might illustrate an increase in the numbers of radiographers at Westwick Hospital over a two-year period.

Table 5.3 Pictogram: example one

Numbers of radiographers	
1988	***
1990	*****

Key * = 5 radiographers

2. Values are not represented accurately by each symbol but an impression is given. An example of this type of pictogram might illustrate an increase in admissions to a medical ward in the period from January to April 19XX.

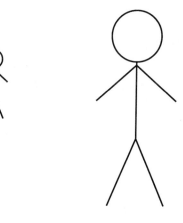

January 19XX   April 19XX

Figure 5.6 Pictogram: example two.

Percentages

Earlier in this chapter we discussed relative frequencies and referred to calculating percentages, assuming this to be a familiar process. We then went on the summarize how to make a pie chart: once again, the concept of a value being proportional to 100 and expressed as a percentage was used. It is also worth noting that this familiar concept can be useful in its own right as a summarizing device for presenting information. For instance, the implication of a statement may not be clear immediately but it can be clarified by giving a percentage value to the data being quoted.

For example, in a study that sampled opinions about the service offered to in-patients by a local hospital, 21 patients out of a group of 200 said they disliked being treated by student therapists. This statement might not have an immediate impact but as a percentage it can be visualized more easily: 10.5% of the sample did not like being treated by students.

Unfortunately the use of percentages can be very misleading. Suppose you were told that 50% of the patients surveyed disliked their therapists. Would you be shocked? Suppose you learned later that the sample in question consisted of four patients and therefore two of these had said that they disliked their therapists. Would that information have the same effect as the '50%' given to you originally? To avoid creating false impressions, it is always wise to give both the actual numbers and their percentage values.

As an example, here are some of the results from a study by Connolly *et al.* (1990) on the use of hoists. There were 134 replies to the circulated questionnaire. The results were summarized as: 'Sixty-five nurses (49%) had received no instruction in the principles of hoist use and 59 (44%) had not been taught to use their ward hoist. Eighty-seven reported that their instruction had been inadequate or nonexistent.'

5.3.2 Summary statistics

It may be necessary to condense data even further into fewer numbers that will still give an overall picture of the research findings. Two statistics used to summarize frequency distributions are:

1. measures of central tendency
2. measures of dispersion.

Measures of central tendency

These statistics express the most typical scores in a distribution. There are three measures of central tendency: the MEAN, the MEDIAN and the MODE. These measures provide us with information about the location of our observations.

The mean

This is probably the most familiar of all statistics and is often known as the arithmetic mean or 'the average'. However, it is inappropriate to limit the word 'average' to the mean because the median and the mode can also justifiably be described in this way. The mean (x) is the sum of all the observations (Σ) divided by the number of the observations (n). It can be expressed as, and calculated by using, a formula that looks like:

$$\bar{x} = \frac{x}{n}$$

Consider a practical example. Suppose the marks gained by a group of therapists (Group S) in an orthotics practical test were as follows:

9, 5, 2, 3, 7, 7, 6, 3, 7, 1
Number of therapists $n = 10$
Sum of scores $= 50$

The mean can be calculated using the formula and substituting the values given above

$$\bar{x} = \frac{x}{n} = \frac{50}{10} = 5$$

Although the mean can always be calculated accurately, it is open to influence by unusual or extreme scores.

The median

This is the middle observation or the observation with the same number of other observations above and below it. It is found, for a small number of scores, by putting all the observations in rank order and finding the central observation. For an ODD number of values, this is achieved by identifying the one in the middle. With an EVEN number of values, it is necessary to take the MEAN value of the middle two scores: in other words, the median lies halfway between the middle two scores of an even number of observations.

Starting with our raw data:

9, 5, 2, 3, 7, 7, 6, 3, 7, 1
these are placed in rank order, giving us
1, 2, 3, 3, 5, 6, 7, 7, 7, 9

Since $n = 10$ (an even number), the middle values (5 and 6) are identified and the mean of these is worked out:

$$\textbf{median} = 5 + 6 = \frac{11}{2} = \textbf{5.5}$$

The mode
The mode is the value that occurs most often or the 'most fashionable one'. In our example the mode is 7 and the distribution can be said to be UNIMODAL as there is only one mode. Where there are two modes, the distribution is said to be BIMODAL.

If Group S of therapists had shown the following scores

9, 5, 2, 3, 7, 7, 6, 2, 8, 1

there would have been two modes, because the scores of 2 and 7 each occur with the same frequency (twice in each case). Where there are more than two modes, the distribution is MULTIMODAL and it is usual to decide that there is no true mode at all.

Let us now return to the idea of a NORMAL DISTRIBUTION, mentioned earlier and discussed further in section 5.4.2. With a normal distribution, the frequency polygon has a characteristic 'bell-shaped curve' illustrated in Figure 5.7. This curve is arranged symmetrically on either side of the mean score. The median and the mode also have the same value as the mean. As any distribution moves away from the norm, the frequency polygon changes its shape to become 'skewed' to one side or the other of the midpoint of the normal distribution curve. The set of scores is then said to be **positively** or **negatively skewed**.

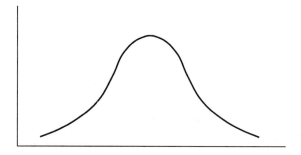

Figure 5.7 Normal distribution curve.

Measures of dispersion

It is quite feasible for measures of central tendency, as discussed above, to be the same for two sets of data which vary enormously in their distribution. So it is important to have some idea of the spread of the observations or the amount of variation there is within any set of observations. In other words, we need to know whether observations are clustered together or whether they are widely dispersed. To meet this need, the RANGE of the raw scores and their deviation from their mean value can be used.

Range
Range is the simplest measure of variation in any set of observations. It can either be quoted in terms of the highest and lowest figures or expressed as the difference between these extreme observations.

Range = largest observation − smallest observation

For Group S therapists, the range is 1 to 9 or a difference of 8.

Consider another example. Suppose that we wanted to compare the orthotics test results for Group S with those obtained by the previous set (Group R). The results for Group R were:

5, 4, 6, 5, 5, 5, 6, 4, 5, 5

The number of subjects (n) remains as ten and the sum of scores is still 55. The mean for this group would be 5, which is the same as for Group S. Thus if we were only to consider the mean, we would suppose the two groups had achieved the same results. However, the range for Group R is 4 to 6 or a difference of 2: this indicates a much closer clustering of the individual results. We can now see clearly that although the mean value of the scores is the same, in Group S there is a greater spread of results than there is in Group R.

There is one situation in which the range of a set of observations is not particularly useful: this is when the smallest and the largest observations are extreme and each is a long way from the next score in the set. Under these conditions, quoting the range does not give us any idea of the spread of values lying between the highest score and the lowest. A better measure of the spread of scores would be their variance or deviation.

Variance
Variance is measured in terms of the deviation of observations from their mean. Deviation is small when observations are located close to their mean and is large if observations are widely scattered. The variation (written as S) is the average of the squares of the differences between each score and the mean of the whole set of scores. It has the formula:

$$S^2 = \frac{\Sigma (x - \bar{x})^2}{(n - 1)}$$

where n = the number of observations or scores

$\bar{x}$ = the mean value of these observations

$x - \bar{x}$ represents the difference between each observation and the mean value.

The denominator $(n - 1)$ is used as this gives a better estimate of the variance of the total population. This number is included in the calculation as an indicator of the DEGREES OF FREEDOM. Readers who would like to know more about the background of this formula are directed to one of the statistical textbooks in the reference list, particularly Siegel and Castellan (1988) and Kirkwood (1988).

Standard deviation

The standard deviation (SD or σ) is the square root of the variance. This statistic reflects the amount by which each score differs from, or is scattered about, the mean. It is therefore a measure of the average dispersion of the variable being investigated. The SD shows the extent of possible error that would be made if the mean alone were to be used to interpret any set of data. We can consider the SD to be the partner of the mean. The mean gives an 'average' score while the SD provides an 'average' deviation from that mean score. It is the most powerful measure of dispersion.

The formula for calculating the SD is:

$$SD = \sqrt{\frac{\Sigma (x - \bar{x})^2}{n}}$$

Let us calculate the SD for the data we have for Group S therapists. Remember that the value of x is 5 for these scores:

Table 5.4 Example of test scores for therapists

Subject no.	Test score	$x - \bar{x}$	$(x - x)^2$
1	9	4	16
2	5	0	0
3	2	−3	9
4	3	−2	4
5	7	2	4
6	7	2	4
7	6	1	1
8	3	−2	4
9	7	2	4
10	1	−4	16
			62

$$SD = \sqrt{\frac{\Sigma (x - \bar{x})^2}{n}}$$

$$= \sqrt{\frac{62}{10}} = \sqrt{6.2} = 2.49$$

We have seen that a small standard deviation indicates that scores do not vary greatly around their mean while a large one suggests a wide dispersion. It is also worth noting that, where observations have a normal distribution, a subset of scores covered by one standard deviation above the mean and one standard deviation below it (expressed as $x \pm 1$ SD) would include 68% of all observations in the set while $x \pm 2$ SD would include 95% and $x \pm 3$ SD would include 97% of those observations.

Semi-interquartile range
Finally, the median has a counterpart which can be used to show the dispersion of a set of scores. This is known as the SEMI-INTERQUARTILE RANGE. To understand how this measure is derived, we need to look again at the example set of scores for Group S after we had set them in rank order and calculated their median score. The vertical line between 5 and 6 shows where the median score would lie: this line divides the set of scores into two equal halves, each with five scores in it.

$$\downarrow \qquad \downarrow$$
$$1, 2, 3, 3, 5, | 6, 7, 7, 7, 9$$

We can now find the quartile scores by selecting the central one in each half. These would be 3 for the quartile below the median and 7 for the quartile above it. These are expressed as Q1 and Q3 respectively.

The formula for the semi-quartile range is written as:

$$\frac{1}{2}(Q3 - Q1)$$

For our set of scores, the semi-quartile range is:

$$\frac{1}{2}(7 - 3) = \frac{4}{2} = 2$$

Rather like the low and high standard deviations we considered earlier, a low semi-quartile range (SI range) indicates that the observations are clustered closely around the median, while a large SI range shows that they are more widely dispersed.

Throughout this section, we have explored the possibilities of using graphic and summary statistics to present information. All these forms of display and measurement allow us to describe our findings effectively, but none of them can enable us to move beyond descriptive statements about what we have collected. In some cases, however, we may want to make predictions based on our investigations: that is, we may have a need to generalize the results. To do this, we would have to turn to the sort of analysis made possible by inferential statistics.

5.4 INFERENTIAL STATISTICS

5.4.1 Introduction

> The theory of statistics is complex but so is the theory behind how a record-player works. We do not need to understand how it works: we only need to know how to switch it on and off.
>
> Jolley (1991)

Consider: if we wanted to find the answer to the question 'What is the mean length of time for which a patient with a Colles fracture is followed up after the plaster is removed?' we would have to collect data from a sample of cases and DESCRIBE the situation at the hospital concerned (relying on descriptive statistics).

However, if we wanted to compare the differences in follow-up at two hospitals, we would need to make inferences from the data (relying on inferential statistics). Or we may know that treatment X was successful in improving the self-care ability of ten patients with multiple sclerosis (MS) and would like to know whether it could be successful for all patients with the same diagnosis. In order to make such a prediction, we need to employ **inferential statistics**, because they enable us to draw inferences from the data collected and therefore to make generalizations.

Principles and concepts of inferential statistics

> The procedures of statistical inference introduce order into any attempt to draw conclusions from the evidence by providing samples . . . statistical tests determine whether, from the evidence we collect, we can have confidence in what we conclude about the larger group from which only a few subjects were sampled.
>
> Siegel and Castellan (1988: 2)

Remembering the metaphor about using a record player without mastering all the details of its mechanical and electrical parts (Jolley, 1991), how much do we need to know about inferential statistics to allow us to 'switch on' the tests that have been developed to bring order into the interpretation of our work? As a first step towards confidence, it is worth exploring some of the words that are used to represent the ideas and rules underlying the tests that are used most often.

Terminology

Over the years, experts have developed and refined a large number of standardized calculations or tests. These can be used to check the extent to which we can draw general conclusions about the data we have collected. In doing so, these statistical experts have also developed special, clear terms for the key concepts that underlie their testing procedures. We need to define the more common of these terms before exploring any of the tests that we might choose.

5.4.2 Samples and populations

Earlier, a sample was defined as a representative subset drawn from a total population. When it comes to testing the legitimacy of any claims we make about our data, **statistics** refer to **samples** while **parameters** relate to **populations**. Castle (1977: 75) suggests an easy way to recall this. You need only remember:

S to S and P to P.

The subjects involved in a study are the SAMPLE but their overall group is a POPULATION. In diagrammatic form, that is:

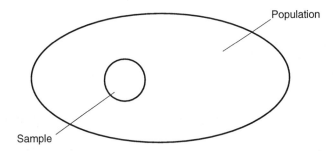

Figure 5.8 Relationship of a sample to a population.

PARAMETERS can be defined as 'measurable characteristics of a case being considered' (*Oxford Concise Dictionary*). In the conventions of statistics, the case being considered is held to be the population from which a sample has been taken. Therefore samples only provide us with estimates about the parameters of their overall group or population. Even if sampling has been carried out correctly, there is a possibility that the sample is not fully representative of the whole population. Thus there is a risk of SAMPLING ERROR. By using inferential statistics, the extent of this error can be estimated and suitable corrections can be made.

Frequency distributions

Earlier in this chapter we introduced the concept of frequencies and touched on the allied concept of normal distribution. It is useful statistically to understand how data are normally distributed because if we understand the normal situation we can make some predictions based on the data we collect. Indeed, some statistical tests rely entirely on the assumption that data are always normally distributed. An illustration of NORMAL DISTRIBUTION which is often used by statisticians is that of the height of any population: if you were to plot the height of every individual in the UK you would produce a graph like this:

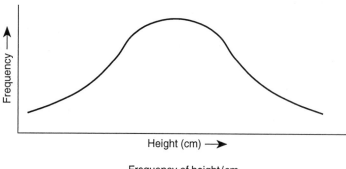

Frequency of height/cm

Figure 5.9 Frequency distribution: normal distribution curve.

The normal distribution is a theoretical distribution assumed for measurements: it allows us to make useful statements of probability. Its curve as a frequency polygon is known as **normal** or **Gaussian**, after a German mathematician called Carl Gauss who described it in 1795. It has the following characteristics:

- The curve is symmetrically 'bell'-shaped. The contour of the bell depends on the variance of the population.

- It is symmetrical on either side of the mean: that is, there are as many spaces to the right of the mean as there are to the left of it. The mean, mode and median are on the same point of the distribution.

- The ends of the curve never touch the horizontal (X) axis. There is thus a small chance of obtaining a very low or a very high score (the curve is ASYMPTOTIC).

- The curve is continuous.

If a distribution is symmetrical, when you draw a line down the centre each half is a mirror image of the other. Both the sample and the whole population should fall into a normal distribution. Where the distribution moves away from the 'normal', the shape of the distribution curve provides valuable information about the data being studied.

Skewness

A distribution is said to be skewed if frequencies are clustered towards one end. Such a distribution can also be said to be asymmetrical. When a distribution is skewed, the mean, mode and median do not share the same value. A distribution may be positively or negatively skewed.

POSITIVELY skewed or skewed TO THE LEFT: a distribution is said to be positively skewed when the largest proportion of data fall below the mean. Such skewness might occur in the results of a difficult examination (Figure 5.10).

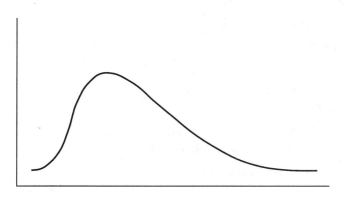

Figure 5.10 Positively skewed distribution curve.

NEGATIVELY skewed or skewed TO THE RIGHT. A distribution is said to be negatively skewed when the largest proportion of the data fall above the mean. This might happen in the results of an easy examination (Figure 5.11).

Skewness is important as it affects the accuracy of statistical analysis and therefore it must be taken into consideration in mathematical equations. Remember, if a distribution is skewed, the mean, mode and median do not share the same value. The median is a valuable indicator of central tendency when a distribution is skewed.

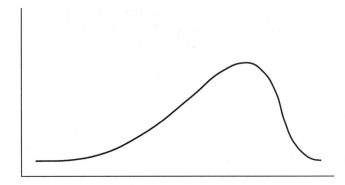

Figure 5.11 Negatively skewed distribution curve.

5.4.3 Probability and significance

These two terms are functionally interdependent. They may be seen as the key concepts supporting any interpretations and conclusions we make once our data have been analysed and tested.

The **probability** of an event or observation refers to the amount of certainty we have that it will or will not happen. Between these two extremes, there is the position that it could have happened as a result of chance alone. In statistics, probability (p) is expressed as a value between 0 and 1, where:

0 represents an event that **is certain NOT to occur**
1 represents an event that **IS certain to occur**.

If we take examples from real life, the probability of every live person dying eventually would be written as p = 1. On the other hand, the probability of someone breathing permanently under water, like a fish, would be written as p = 0. On the continuum that lies between p = 1 to p = 0, those events that cannot be forecast with certainty can be given values reflecting the likelihood of their happening. Where there is no evidence of other cause, an event is said to have a p value of 0.5: that is, it happened by chance. If we extend this logic, we can see that the nearer a p value for any event is to 0, the less likely it is to be due to chance (or the more **significant** it is). In calculating the probability of any event occurring, the following formula is used:

$$p = \frac{\text{number of occurrences}}{\text{total number of possible occurrences}}$$

The most common example given of probability at chance level is that of tossing a coin to achieve heads (HE) rather than tails. This is expressed as:

$$HE = \frac{\text{heads}}{\text{heads and tails}} = \frac{1}{2} + 0.5$$

However, we must notice that the answer is only a probability: we cannot PROVE anything. When we apply this to a well-designed research project with two groups of patients, one given a treatment package and the other not, a difference in their performance at post-test would have to be tested. If the statistical test showed a p value of 0.5, then we would know that the difference between the two groups had happened **by chance** alone. However, if the test were to give a p value **less than 0.5**, we could assume that the treatment had influenced the performance of the group that had received it.

Even when results can be shown to be statistically significant, this is only one of several factors we have to consider. You will have to deal with the issue of the clinical and practical application of your results. If the difference we can make with a change in treatment is small, the cost of adopting a new regime may not be merited.

Significance and levels of significance

> Tests of significance indicate whether the difference between the observed results and those expected from the original hypothesis is likely to have been due to chance.
>
> Ogier (1989: 22)

Once the data have been analysed and results have been processed using an appropriate statistical test, a numerical outcome is produced. This raw outcome, or number, has a level of significance in terms of the test that has been used. The level of the raw outcome can then be checked against the relevant table of significance. Such tables are normally printed in the appendices of textbooks that cover the processes of statistical analysis and interpretation. Several examples of books that introduce people to statistical testing are listed at the end of this book.

The lower the p value, the more likely it is that the results obtained are not due to chance. In other words, the lower the p value, the higher the level of significance. Listed below are some examples illustrating these principles.

When the probability of an event being due to chance alone is **less than** 5 in 1000 this is expressed as

$p < 0.005$ = significant

Even higher levels of significance might be written as:

$p < 0.001$ = more significant (less than 1 in 1000)
and $p < 0.0001$ = very significant (less than 1 in 10 000)

In contrast, when the probability of an event being due to chance alone is **more than** 5 in 10, this is expressed as:

$$p > 0.5 = \text{not significant}$$

Clearly, there are many other levels of significance between the examples given above. It is usual in health-related and social studies to adopt a particular level of significance and to maintain that as the 'gold standard' throughout a project. The choice of a guiding level of significance can vary between styles and settings of research, but very often an acceptable level of significance is agreed as $p = 0.01$ (or $p < 0.02$).

A final word about significance leads on to the matter of using statistical tests to support or reject an hypothesis. The power of tests and the limitations of their interpretation depends to some extent on whether we have anticipated that results will go in one direction or whether we have said that results could go in either of two opposite directions. Since we take no risk if we have no clear expectation of the outcome of our studies, it is not surprising that there is a price to pay for our lack of confidence. For the same raw outcome, the p value for a two-tailed prediction is less significant than it would be for a one-tailed prediction. There are tables of **one-tailed** and **two-tailed probabilities** which have to be consulted after calculating a raw outcome figure. (Once again, it would be wise to refer to an introductory statistics book if you need to explore these mathematical concepts further.)

Correlation

By calculating the **correlation**, we can demonstrate the amount of association, or match, there is between two sets of measurements, scores or observations. There are several ways of testing data for correlation, with limitations of use depending on the type of data under analysis. Generally, the correlation tests are divided into two categories – PARAMETRIC and NON-PARAMETRIC – which apply to ordinal, interval and ratio scale data and to nominal data respectively (see also page 129 below). Tests in both categories lead to a **correlation coefficient** which is expressed by using numbers between $+1$, 0 and -1 to indicate how much correspondence there is between two sets of measurement.

　　0 = there is **no match** between the figures
　+1 = there is a **perfect match** between the figures.

To illustrate this system:

　　0.9 shows a high level of correlation while
　　0.1 indicates practically no correlation.

So far, we have been referring to POSITIVE correlations, for example, where the heights and weights of a group of people have been compared and it has been found that, in general, the taller people are also the heavier ones. To complete the picture of correlations, we must now consider situations where there are NEGATIVE associations between two sets of scores. For these situations, a perfect correlation would be expressed as -1. We might find this sort of correlation if we checked the dental health of children and their regular intake of sweets. Here we might find that the children who eat most sweets have the worst dental health.

Before leaving this brief discussion on correlation, it is important to understand that, although a correlation coefficient shows that two sets of measurements have some association, it cannot be used to claim that one measured attribute CAUSES the other. It can only show that these attributes COEXIST.

5.4.4 Choice of tests

Without the advantage of years of research experience and faced with a plethora of available tests, how do you decide which ones to use? Put another way, how do you know which tests can be applied to your data and which are the most appropriate when it comes to interpreting them? At this point, I make no apology for reminding you that we have advised you on two occasions that no research study should be started without asking an expert in statistics to guide you. As long as you have planned your data collection knowing how you are going to analyse it, the decisions on suitable tests will have been taken at the beginning of your project. Nevertheless, it is probably helpful to summarize the factors that have to be considered when you are debating which type of test to use.

Considerations limiting the choice of tests

The type of measurement used
Nominal scale data require non-parametric tests, while ordinal and interval scale data can be analysed appropriately by either parametric or non-parametric tests. The choice between these two types of test depends on the distribution of the observations and the extent to which this tallies with the population from which the sample is taken. Because there is greater power in parametric tests, these are used in preference to non-parametric ones whenever possible. To analyse true ratio scale data, parametric tests are used.

The number of groups used and their inter-relationships
Particular tests are recommended for one-sample, two-samples and three-or-more (k) samples involved in a study. It is also possible to use tests that

have been developed for analysing data from related or independent samples.

The avoidance of sampling bias

Some tests can only be used if the inclusion of one subject in a study did not prejudice the chances of inclusion for any other member of the total population under investigation. In general, a sample achieved by random selection gives the greatest choice of appropriate tests.

These and other considerations are fully covered in Reid and Boore (1987). If you are about to discuss your study plans with an expert, you will probably find it helpful to spend some time becoming familiar with the names and purposes of some of the more commonly used tests. Remember, whatever you do, decide on the tests you are going to use **before** you collect any data.

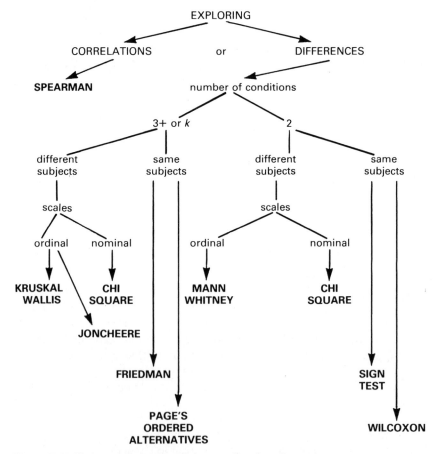

Figure 5.12 Tests applied to conditions and scales of measurement.

Referring to Figure 5.12 you will see the names of some of the commonly used statistical tests. The summary below highlights the reasons for applying each of them, shown in answer to general research questions. In some cases, a familiar scenario is used to illustrate the application of a test.

Spearman's rho: correlation indicator
This tests whether there is a clear association between two sets of scores for the same individuals. Each set of scores is ranked and the agreement or correlation of the ranks per person is tested. Within professional education, we might want to see whether there is any correlation between performance in theoretical examinations and fieldwork achievement.

Chi Square test and Mann Whitney U test
Both these tests can be used to indicate whether there is a significant difference between the scores of two unrelated samples. To illustrate the framework of a Chi square analysis, let us consider that two groups of stroke patients, each numbering 30 people, were observed under two conditions. Group A received daily speech and language re-education, Group B had no communication therapy. Using an assessment of spoken English, all subjects were rated after six weeks as having improved (I) or having not improved (NI). Table 5.5 below shows the results, set in a two-by-two grid.

Table 5.5 Two-by-two grid showing test results for patients

	Improved	*Not improved*	*Total*
A Speech and language re-education	18	12	30
B No communication therapy	25	5	30
Total	43	17	60

The *Mann Whitney U test* treats the scores from two independent samples by setting them in rank order. The full range of ranks is allocated for both groups as a whole and then the ranking of people in each group is identified. The sum of the ranks for the treatment group are checked against the sum of the ranks for the control group. The test identifies which group has predominately low ranks and which group has mainly high ranks.

Sign test and Wilcoxon test
These tests are applied to two sets of related scores. The Sign test is based on the DIRECTION of the differences between two measures. It is a

particularly useful test when data cannot be quantified in themselves but it is possible to say that in each pair of observations (x and y), one is greater than the other. In this situation, each subject is used as his/her own control. Data are compared and allocated a 'sign', that is:

where x is greater than y a positive sign ($+$) is allocated
where x is less than y a negative sign ($-$) is allocated.

For example, a treatment unit was asked to investigate the therapist and client contribution to planning treatment goals. This was explored by asking representatives of therapists and clients to rate the control assumed (dominance) by each 'player' in the decisions being taken about treatment goals. Using therapist/client pairs, the therapists rated clients and their own influence while the clients rated therapists and their own influence. The results were coded in terms of client influence as:

$+$ if the client should have greater influence than the therapist, according to the therapist
$-$ if the client should have less influence than the therapist, according to the therapist.

The Wilcoxon Signed rank test is more powerful than the Sign test because it uses the SIZE (magnitude) of differences as well as their DIRECTION (positive or negative). The size of the differences is indicated by ranking the differences for the combined scores.

Tests for different subjects and same subjects with three or more (k) conditions

In anticipation that you are more likely to use two groups than k groups when you are designing your first study, not all the possibilities shown on Figure 5.13 are outlined here. Full details and explanations of the Kruskal-Wallis one-way analysis of variance, the Chi Square test for data entered in a $2 \times k$ grid, the Joncheere test for ordered alternatives and Page's test for ordered alternatives can be found in Siegel and Castellan (1988). Figure 5.12 indicates which of these tests can be applied to related and unrelated data for several conditions of observation.

The Friedman Two-way analysis of variance by ranks Some comments on this test are made here to illustrate the possibilities of observing and comparing the results under several conditions. For example, you might wish to explore the progress of patients, matched for age, sex, diagnosis and length of time since onset of disorder, under four different treatment procedures. Provided that you have been able to record observations on at least an ordinal scale, the data from these matched samples could be tested by Friedman's analysis of variance (Friedman's ANOVA).

Parametric and non-parametric tests

These two classes of statistical tests have been mentioned several times: you have probably gathered by now that the differences between them stem from the conditions under which each can be used. Each statistical test is based on a model and has a measurement requirement, which are called collectively the 'assumptions' of the test.

> The test is valid under certain conditions and the model and the measurement requirement specify these conditions. Sometimes we are able to test whether the conditions of a particular statistical model are met, but more often we have to assume that they are met.
>
> Siegel and Castellan (1988)

The stronger the assumptions of a test, the greater is its power and the more confident we can be in reaching conclusions. Conversely, the weaker the test assumptions, the smaller is its power, leaving us with very general conclusions. Parametric tests assume, at least, a sample population that has a normal distribution of the variable being measured, the use of ordinal, interval or ratio scale measurement and independence of observations. Where two groups of subjects are under observation, there must be similarity of variance in the groups.

> Parametric tests are those which are limited by a necessary adherence to certain underlying assumptions, mainly concerned with the characteristics of the population distribution from which the sample was drawn.
>
> Wright and Fowler (1986: 46)

Non-parametric tests, in contrast, have less extensive assumptions, so they are also known as 'distribution free' tests. They do not oblige you to check the characteristics of your subject groups with as much stringency as parametric tests. Because they are not as sensitive, they do not have the same power as their parametric equivalents when they are applied to the same data. Having made these formal comparisons, it is worth noting that if you are not sure whether your data can meet the conditions for a parametric test, you can err on the side of caution and choose a non-parametric test.

5.5 USE OF A COMPUTER

> The computer will probably do at least as much to change the nature and future of the world as the wheel or the printing press.
>
> Goldstone (1983: 152)

Without any doubt, using a computer in the analysis of research data makes it possible to carry out detailed procedures reliably and very quickly. It is extremely important to check that all the data have been entered accurately. Many therapists are already familiar with the computers used in their daily work and will recognize what I am saying. Basically, the computer is a moron: it has no discretion and will do EXACTLY what you ask it to do but no more. If you use a statistical test that is not appropriate for your data, the computer will not alert you to the error in your ways. A student recently coded all the men in her study as 1 and all the women as 2. From the computer analysis, she was able to tell me that the mean of the sexes was 1.5. She did not appreciate initially that this finding was meaningless and argued that the mean must be correct because that was the result provided by the computer. It was not until she tried to make sense of the data in real terms that she realized the problem.

Remember the saying: 'Garbage in, garbage out' with regard to the analysing of results. In other words, if you put meaningless, incomprehensible information into a computer, that is exactly what you will get out of it.

If you are going to use a computer to analyse your data, this must be considered at a very early stage in your planning. All necessary arrangements must be made well in advance and you will still need to consult an expert in statistics for advice on the choice of suitable tests. Once the basic choices have been made, there are several software packages, such as SPSSX and Mintiab, which can be used. It is very important that you maintain credibility in analysing your data and do not process them in a misleading way. It is helpful to consider the following five points suggested by Huff (1954: 110) to check whether the statistical processes that have been used are sound, as well as the interpretation.

1. WHO says so? You need to look for conscious and unconscious bias as well as considering the standing and reputation of the researcher.
2. HOW do they know? Check the sample used in the study, the method used to obtain the findings and the power of the study.
3. What is MISSING? Be careful of averages and percentages used instead of figures. Remember that missing information could account for the results that have been obtained. For example, if more patients are being discharged from an orthopaedic ward since the appointment of an extra therapist, but the report does not mention the introduction of new surgical techniques within the period of the study, this improved discharge rate might be attributed to the increase in staff numbers alone.
4. Did someone CHANGE the subject(s) being considered? This may seem to be an unlikely action, but it can happen, either because data have been confused at some stage of the analysis/interpretation or because some cases being discussed are not the same as others within the study.

5. Does it make SENSE? It is sound advice to use commonsense when all else fails. Remember that extrapolations are useful but that in most cases, predictions or trends for the future can really be no more than educated guesses (Huff, 1954: 123).

It is also important to be familiar with the responsibilities that researchers take on when they decide to use computerized recording systems. It is not enough to meet professional, ethical and moral expectations alone. All researchers who hold and analyse any data on a computer about the people who take part in their studies are also bound by legal requirements. These are laid down in an Act of Parliament.

Data Protection Act 1984

Any personal details on subjects which are stored on a computer are covered by the regulations of this Act. If you are planning to use a computer to record and analyse your data, you should study the Act in detail, but the main principles are:

- Personal data shall be processed fairly and lawfully
- Personal data shall be held only for one or more specified lawful purpose
- Personal data held for any purpose shall not be used or disclosed in any manner incompatible with that purpose
- Personal data held for any purpose shall be adequate, relevant and not excessive in relation to that purpose
- Personal data shall be accurate and, where necessary, kept up to date
- An individual shall be entitled to, on request and for a fee, a copy of the personal data held about themselves and, where appropriate, to have such data corrected or erased
- Appropriate security measures shall be taken against unauthorized access to, or alteration, disclosure or destruction of, personal data and against accidental loss or destruction of personal data.

5.6 DRAWING CONCLUSIONS

Once your data has been analysed, whether by computer software or by manual calculations, the final task in every research project is to interpret the findings and the evidence they provide to support or refute the answers you have been seeking. In some cases, where a formal hypothesis was made at the beginning of a study, the researcher has to weigh the evidence and decide whether or not the null hypothesis can be rejected. In other cases, a trend can be demonstrated, a significant correlation is shown or an unexpected relationship between variables seems likely to stimulate further studies before confident conclusions can be made.

It is at this stage that discussion of the findings with interested colleagues can again be a good investment of your time. This sort of discussion will help you to sharpen up your thinking about the results and will identify the real and admissible conclusions lurking among your impressions of the whole study. If the statistical analysis has been a somewhat daunting operation, it is worth while to meet with your statistical adviser to find out their views on the results. They will be more familiar than you are with interpreting and applying the probabilities you have read from the tables of significance.

Whatever the outcome of your research, it will be important as you make your conclusions to recall all the stages in the research and to link them, and your results, with the ideas and evidence derived from your literature search. Remember that you will move on to writing up your work and the claims you make in your conclusions will pull together all the details you want to share with your colleagues.

STATISTICS: FURTHER READING

Bayliss, D. (1983a) Statistics for nurses 1: Collection and presentation of data. *Nursing Times*, **79** (43), 47–50.

Bayliss, D. (1983b) Statistics for nurses 2: Mode, median, mean: range and standard deviation. *Nursing Times*, **79** (44), 31–3.

Bayliss, D. (1983c) Statistics for nurses 3: Correlation and regression. *Nursing Times*, **79** (5), 25–7.

Jolley, J. (1991) Computing in practice: Using statistics. *Nursing Times*, 19 June, **87** (25), 57–9.

Kirkwood, B.R. (1988) *Essentials of Medical Statistics*, Blackwell Scientific, Oxford.

Rowntree, D. (1981) *Statistics Without Tears: A Primer for Non-Mathematicians*, Penguin Books, Harmondsworth.

Siegal, S. and Castellan, N.J. (1988) *Non-parametric Systems for the Behavioural Sciences*, McGraw-Hill, New York.

SUPPLIERS OF PUBLISHED AND STANDARDIZED TESTS

NFER-Nelson
Marketing Services Department
FREEPOST, Windsor, Berkshire, SL4 1BU

Psychological Corporation
24–28 Oval Road
London NW1 7DX

Writing up

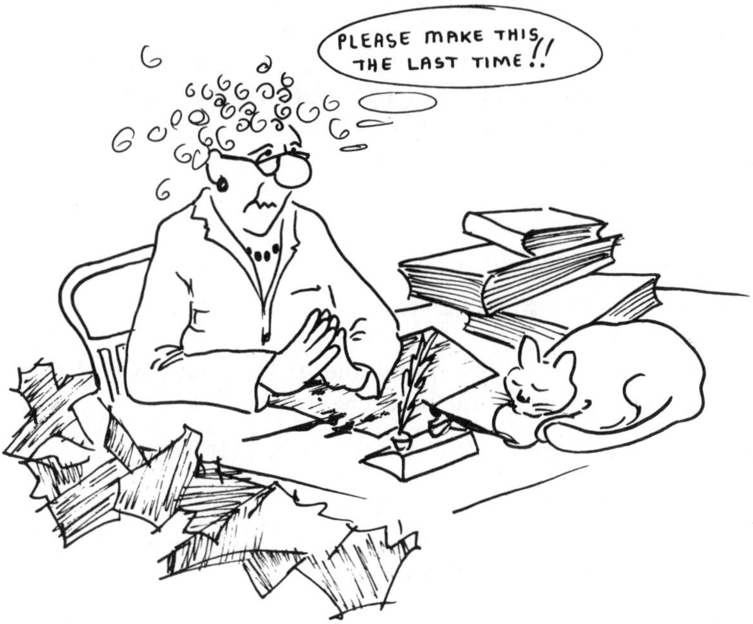

Figure 6.1 Writing up.

Good scientific journalese comes with practice.

Hicks (1988: 235)

Researchers should assume that they have principal responsibility for dissemination and ensure that their results are accessible to the widest possible audience.

Richardson, Jackson and Sykes (1990)

For many researchers, writing-up is the worst part of the whole research process. They view this aspect with very negative feelings and often delay starting. However, I think that this is one of the most important parts of research. If you do not commit your results to paper, you will limit the number of professional colleagues who can learn from your study. You may waste valuable information which could have enormous benefits for others. So communicating the results of a study is an important part of the whole research process.

6.1 ESSENTIALS FOR WRITING UP

When it comes to making the best possible use of a chance to **communicate** by writing, most of us use a mixture of personal inspiration, supporting 'tools' and suitable surroundings that we choose for ourselves. However, there are some basic facilities that are essential for good writing (items 1–3 below) and others that depend on whether we have a choice between manual composition or word processing.

Minimum requirements for writing-up

1. Access to the following books:

   - An English dictionary to check the spelling and usage of words (for example is it therapeutic practice or practise?)

   - A medical dictionary to check the spelling of medical terms

   - *Roget's Thesaurus*

   - A grammar textbook. My personal favourite is a book by Temple (1978) which is very easy to read.

   Before you moan at the latter, think about your knowledge regarding the use of paragraphs, whether to use a colon or a semi-colon and when to put an apostrophe before or after an 's'. Remember if your grammar and English are poor, it will reflect badly on the entire study. If the presentation is careless, it might suggest that there is a similar carelessness in the research project itself. Apley (1976) commented that 'good grammar . . . is good manners in writing'. Calnan and Barabas (1973: 97) believe 'Bad writing is a slovenly habit.'
2. A room that is well lit, adequately heated and ventilated and free from distraction.
3. A comfortable chair and a table that does not move when you write.
4. Any other relevant material, data, articles or books.

5. For manual composition, lots of paper and a good quality pen. Writing with a cheap blotchy pen makes the whole task even harder.
6. For word processing, familiarity with and unlimited access to a word processor or computer with flexible software.

Writing-up is a self-discipline and you must be strict to work for several hours at a stretch. Even if the process does not come together as you planned, use the time to revise important articles, jot down ideas and outline sketches.

When you begin to draft your write-up, number the pages as you go along. Leave wide margins and, if possible, only write on alternate lines; this makes corrections and additions easier to insert. If you are using a word processor or computer, work in double spacing and do not make use of 'headers' and 'footers' until the first draft has been composed. **Remember to save** your work at least every two pages. It is also important to make a back-up copy of your document(s) at the end of each session on the computer.

NEVER show a first draft to anyone. It is for your eyes only and needs more work before you are in a position to ask anyone else to make comments. If you ask people to read your write-up too early, they will lose enthusiasm later and you will be depressed by their feedback. Early drafts are attempts to sort out what should be included. Subsequent drafts tidy up the material and final drafts are the 'icing': that is, they are for polishing up the material to the highest possible standard. Wainwright (1984: 48) recommends leaving at least 24 hours between writing a draft and revising it in order to achieve clarity.

When you are writing, avoid:

- poor English and incorrect grammar

- bad punctuation

- jargon

- pomposity

- verbosity

- colloquialisms

- abbreviations (your readers will hate them).

Make sure you check:

- spelling

- flow and continuity

- labelling of all diagrams, figures and tables

- the tenses of verbs: these should usually be in the past tense.

Wainwright (1984: 57) has suggested some amusing and excellent tips for writers. These include:

- do not use no double negatives

- verbs has to agree with their subject

- avoid commas, that are not necessary

- if you reread your work, you will find on rereading that a great deal of repetition can be avoided by editing

- it is incumbent upon us to avoid archaic words.

Another interesting author who offers ideas on the use and misuse of words is Sternberg (1988: 75). Dealing with the word 'only', he illustrates how its position in a sentence can alter the meaning.

> I will only treat the patient in my office tomorrow.
> I will treat the only patient in my office tomorrow.
> I will treat the patient only in my office tomorrow.
> I will treat the patient in my office only tomorrow.

6.1.1 Gunning's Fog Index

Gunning's Fog Index (Gunning, 1968) is an excellent way of assessing the readability of your text in terms of its 'fogginess'. The score indicates the amount of schooling someone needs in order to read your text with ease.
    In order to calculate a fog score:

1. Count a sample of 100 words.
2. Find the average number of words per sentence = X.
3. Count the number of words in the sample with three or more syllables = Y.

    DO NOT count words:

    - which begin with a capital letter

    - which are combinations of short words (e.g. over-heated)

    - that have been made into three syllables by ending in '-ed' or '-es' (e.g. collected, provided, approaches)
4. Calculate the score thus:

$$(X + Y) \times 0.4 = \text{FOG INDEX}$$

A fog index of below 5 is very easy reading whereas an index of above 17 is extremely difficult. Where the fog index exceeds 10, the text is placing an obstacle around the ideas it is trying to convey.
    Compare the fog scores for the following:

The Bible	6.5
Daily Mirror	9.2
Government circular	23.2

As many medical terms are polysyllabic, the Fog Index can be difficult to apply in paramedical literature. However, it provides a valuable rule of thumb for general writing style.

6.2 WRITING A THESIS

A copy of the guidelines provided by the university or institution where you are registered should be read carefully. If such guidelines have not been provided, write to the academic registrar and ask for a copy. This document should be followed exactly in preference to any other publications. Any difficulties that arise from it should be clarified with a supervisor or mentor.

There will be some differences between institutions about the exact layout of dissertations. There will obviously also be differences between dissertations by virtue of the fact that they are being submitted for different qualifications. However, by convention, the most widely used layout is based on the IMRAD structure. That is:

I–ntroduction
M–ethod
R–esults
A–nd
D–iscussion

Bradford-Hill (1965) felt that writing should answer the questions 'Why did you start, what did you do, what answer did you get, and what does it mean anyway?' The IMRAD structure relates directly to this.

Why? – Introduction
What? – Method
Answer? – Results
Meaning? – Discussion

Although this is the order the majority of dissertations follow, it is not necessarily the order in which they are written. Indeed, many researchers advocate beginning not at the beginning, but with the method and results. These are considered easier to write as they are factual sections. As they take shape, they will help to clarify points that need to be raised in the introduction, discussion and conclusions. Another benefit of writing in this way is that you can attempt to avoid wandering off course, particularly in the introduction and discussion, as many individuals are inclined to do.

The dissertation will usually include:

Title
This should be informative without being verbose.

Acknowledgements
It is polite to acknowledge the help provided by others during the research. This help may be in the form of finance, advice, practical assistance or moral support.

Contents
The contents of each chapter should be listed with a page reference. This should be followed by references and appendices if applicable.

If tables or illustrations appear in the dissertation, they should be listed separately under the headings of:

● List of tables.

● List of illustrations, to include maps, diagrams, pictures and photographs.

Abstract
As the abstract is a summary of the whole study, it is usually written last. It should include the aim of the study, the method of research and the main results obtained. The maximum length is approximately 500 words.

The abstract is usually the first part of the study to be read, so it is important that it is accurate and interesting. If the abstract is poor, it will reduce the enthusiasm of the reader (or more importantly the examiner) to continue reading.

Introduction
The introduction sets the scene for the dissertation and answers the question 'Why?'. Comparisons should be made with other studies in the field and similarities and contrasts drawn. It is not the aim of this section to give a complete historical account of previous work. The introduction may be considered as funnel-shaped. It starts generally and narrows to the specific question in hand.

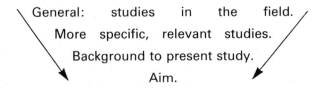

General: studies   in   the   field.
More   specific,   relevant   studies.
Background to present study.
Aim.

Figure 6.2 Funnel-shaped design for the introduction.

Method

This is the 'How?' section. How did you conduct the research? The method section of a thesis is similar to a cookery recipe: it tells you how the research was done in the same way a cookery recipe tells you how to make a sponge pudding. You should cover the research design, your choice of subjects, the questionnaire/interview design, the method of analysis chosen and any other pertinent points in the same way that a recipe lists the ingredients used.

If the methodology chosen is new, or not commonly used in your research area, you should also include some justification for its use. This should include a review of the literature in order to lend credibility to the method you have chosen.

Results

This section is often said to be the easiest to write up as it is factual However, it can be difficult to decide what to include as even the smallest study can generate a lot of information. Raw data should never be presented, for example, the individual scores for each patient obtained in each test. Instead you must try to make sense of the data you obtain and pass a summary of this to the reader.

The information presented should not be biased and the normal values for tests should also be given if the reader is unlikely to know them. No comments on the data should be presented in this section. This is often a common mistake made in writing-up for the first time: only the FACTS appear here.

One final word of caution. Lead the reader through this section as you would lead a blind person through a wood. Introduce what you are presenting initially and accompany each change in direction with an explanation. Guard against presenting a boring mound of information with little apparent rhyme or reason. If the method is the recipe, then the results section is a description of what you found when you opened the oven door.

Discussion

In this section the results are interpreted and comments made in the light of the work that has been discussed in the introduction. This section may be considered an opposite funnel-shape to that in the introduction. Thus:

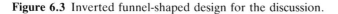

Results of study interpreted.
Results related to other work in area.
General application and relevance of findings.

Figure 6.3 Inverted funnel-shaped design for the discussion.

It is important that the findings of the study are linked to the work of others in the field; comments on similarities and differences should be made and, with the latter, possible explanations offered.

You should also comment on the limitations of the study, particularly any flaws in its methodology. There is more merit in displaying your critical skills by highlighting flaws than in attempting to conceal them. In any case, they are probably obvious to the reader/examiner. Where problems are not so obvious, they should still be mentioned. As Kane (1985: 176) so aptly noted: 'Science advances by explaining what went wrong as well as what went right.'

Conclusions and recommendations (if appropriate)

The main conclusions should be put in a separate section rather than in the discussion. It is important to 'round up' the findings of the research, but this must be done within the constraints and limitations of the study. The majority of research findings merely indicate a trend, not firm facts. The conclusions drawn should be worded very carefully as, indeed, should any recommendations you make. For example, if you found that patients with rheumatoid arthritis (RA) had increased range of movement after using a particular type of orthosis, you could not draw the conclusion 'All patients with RA should be given an orthosis.' Be honest and link this section with what you actually found.

On a lighter note, remember that it is an unwritten tradition that most researchers finish their writing-up by concluding that there is a need for more research in their area.

References

All references mentioned in the study should be listed. Do not try to 'pad out' the study by listing references you have not actually used. This is a cardinal sin. Wherever possible use the primary reference source: that is, try to read the actual reference and not someone else's interpretation of it. Always quote accurately and check your sources when writing-up the reference section.

There are several methods of presentation and it is important to refer to the guidelines provided by the university (or publisher). Where this is not specified, choose one method and keep to it. The main styles are:

The Harvard style

In this system references are given in a list by the author's surname in alphabetical order. They are indicated in the text by the surname of the author and the year of publication. This is the system used in this book.

For example: text: It has been suggested that stroke patients need active leisure participation (Drummond, 1990); or: Drummond (1990) has suggested that stroke patients need active leisure participation. Reference list: Drummond, A. (1990) Leisure activity after stroke. *International Disability Studies*, **12** (4), 157–60.

The Vancouver style

This style is favoured by the International Committee of Medical Journal Editors (1982). Each reference is given a number according to where it appears in the text. When this reference is used, a number appears.

For example, for a reference taken from a journal:

text: Investigations of the leisure pursuits of stroke patients have shown participation in leisure decreases after stroke.[1,2]

Reference list:

1. Sjogren, K. (1982) Leisure after stroke. *Int Rehabil Med*, **4**, 80–7.
2. Feibel, J.H. and Springer, C.J. (1982) Depression and failure to resume social activities after stroke. *Arch Phys Med Rehabil*, **63**, 276–8.

As a personal tip (offered from bitter experience), if you choose this style do not number references until the last draft. If you do begin the numbering process before this, you will find that, as the order of paragraphs changes and further references are inserted, you will end up amazingly confused about who said what and when.

Summary of detailed entries

The format of a JOURNAL reference is usually: surname, initials, year of publication, title, journal, volume, pages. For example: Drummond, A. (1988) Stroke: the impact on the family. Br J Occup Ther, **51** (6), 193–4.

Note that the abbreviations used to indicate journals have been standardized (e.g. Br J Occup Ther for *British Journal of Occupational Therapy*). The standard abbreviations can be found in the *Index Medicus* LIST OF JOURNALS INDEXED, published annually.

The format of a BOOK reference is usually: surname, initial(s), date of publication, title, edition (if relevant), publisher, city of publication, pages (if relevant). For example:

Moffat, D.B. and Mottram, R.F. (1979) *Anatomy and Physiology for Physiotherapists*, Blackwell Scientific Publications, London, pp. 212–18;

Squires, A.J. (ed.) (1988) *Rehabilitation of the Older Patient*, Croom Helm, London.

Reference to a CHAPTER in a book is usually given by author's surname, initial(s), year of publication, in: title, editor (or author) of actual book, its title, publisher, city of publication, pages. For example: Stallworthy, J. (1985) Give a reference, in: Lock, S. (ed.) *How to do it*, (2nd edn) British Medical Association, London, pp. 71–3.

Note the use of punctuation in the examples given above. Before you submit any written material for possible publication, make sure that you have used commas, full stops and recognized abbreviations correctly within your reference list. It will save you the embarrassment of being asked by the editor to put things right.

Where there are more than three authors, the term '*et al.*' (and others) can be used in the text, but the names of all the authors must be listed in the reference section. When there are more than six authors, '*et al.*' can be used after the sixth listed author.

If an article has been accepted for publication but not yet published, it can be referenced as 'in press'. If it has been submitted but not yet accepted, it is 'unpublished observations' or 'accepted for publication'.

Appendices
Notice that the plural is appendices and the singular is appendix. This section should include material which is **relevant** to the study but which is either too long to put in the main body or which would detract from the flow. Examples of material suitable for inclusion as an appendix include a copy of the questionnaire used, details of the format used for interviews or correspondence related to the study.

The most frequently asked question concerning dissertations is 'How long should it be?' Evans (1978) commented 'it should be long enough to ensure adequate presentation of the work but that it should not be artificially lengthened by the inclusion of irrelevant subject matter'.

6.3 WRITING A PAPER

Bradford-Hill (1965: 870) believed that the fundaments of the scientific paper were to communicate what the author thought had been found out and how it had been found. Writing a paper can be difficult because you are expected to condense a wealth of information into a succinct, well-written, informative article. Before the whole idea depresses you too greatly, remember that it is always much easier to condense information than it is to create it.

The general guidelines given under section 6.2 also apply to the preparation of a paper. In particular, the details for compiling references and the ways in which these should be cited in the paper are identical. Decide as early as possible which journal you are aiming to publish in. Each journal has its own 'house style' and has specific guidelines for authors which give the format, length and style of referencing to be used. For example, *Physiotherapy* and *British Journal of Occupational Therapy* both have individual house styles. If the journal does not print this in each issue, you must ask for a copy of the author's guidelines from the editor. Although guidelines are invaluable, there is always a great deal of consideration over the length of a proposed paper. It can be irritating to be told that an article should be long enough to cover the material but this is indeed the case.

When more than one author is involved in a paper, it is also important to decide early who is the first author. Similarly, it is important to decide who should be listed as a co-author. Only individuals who have been involved directly in the research should be named. Other people should be mentioned and thanked individually in the acknowledgements.

The conventional format for an article is the IMRAD structure (section 6.2) although this only covers the most important points. It is usually best to cover one line of thought only in a paper. If you introduce too many aims you will end up with a confused paper which succeeds in saying nothing. Other important issues can be written up in other papers and cross-referenced as necessary.

After your paper has been submitted for publication it will be reviewed by at least two reviewers. It is uncommon to have a paper accepted unconditionally: usually advice is given on rewriting sections or including additional material or omitting irrelevant information. Once such revisions have been made, the article may then be accepted. Do not be upset if a paper is rejected: it happens to everyone at some stage. It may be that your paper is too specialized or unsuitable for the journal you have submitted it to. If this happens, try to get an honest opinion about the problem from the editor.

6.3.1 Proofreading

Only submit what you want to see published. There is some opportunity to change small details after review but proofreading is exactly that: reading the proofs before printing. You may have to pay if you make substantial changes to the script, except where the printer is at fault. It is important that you read the whole article carefully and check it meticulously. Look for mistakes in the spelling of specialized terms, references and in the numbers presented. Avoid mistakes in print by proofreading thoroughly. It is wise to keep a copy of the proofs and the corrections you have made.

Most journals send the proofs with a guide on how to make corrections. The most common are the Standard British instructions for proofreading. See pp. 144–150.

Remember there are often long delays from submission to acceptance of a paper – and indeed from the latter to publication. Smith (1991) gives some explanation for this by providing an insight into the many processes involved in publishing an article in the *Australian Occupational Therapy Journal*. Most major journals have a backlog of papers awaiting comments by reviewers, corrections from authors and preparations for publication.

INSTRUCTION	TEXTUAL MARK	MARGINAL MARK
Correction is concluded	None	/
Leave unchanged	under characters to remain	✓
Remove extraneous marks	Encircle marks to be removed	✗
Push down risen spacing material	Encircle blemish	⊥
Refer to appropriate authority anything of doubtful accuracy	Encircle words affected	(?)
Insert in text the matter indicated in the margin	⅄	New matter followed by: ⅄
Insert additional matter identified by a letter in a diamond	⅄	⅄ Followed by, for example: ◇A
Delete	/ through character(s) or ⊢——⊣ though words to be deleted	♂⁊
Delete and close up	∫ through character or ⊢——⊣ through characters eg character character	
Substitute character or substitute part of one or more word(s)	/ through character or ⊢——⊣ through word(s)	New character or new word(s)

INSTRUCTION	TEXTUAL MARK	MARGINAL MARK
Wrong fount. Replace by character(s) or correct fount	Encircle characters to be changed	(⊗)
Change damaged characters	Encircle character(s) to be changed	✕
Set in or change to italic	——— under character(s) to be set or changed	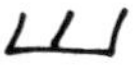 ⎿⎿⏌
Set in or change to capital letters	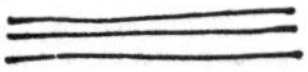 ═══ under character(s) to be set or changed	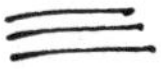 ═
Set in or change to small capital letters	═══ under characters to be set or changed	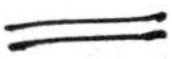 ═
Set in or change to capital letters for initial letters and small capital letters for the rest of the words	 ═ under initial letters and ═══ under the rest of the word(s)	═
Set in or change to bold type	 ∿∿∿ under character(s) to be set or changed	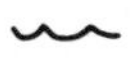 ∿
Set in or change to bold italic type	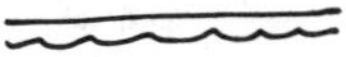 ∿∿∿ under character(s) to be set or changed	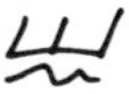 ⎿⎿⏌∿
Change capital letters to lower case letters	Encircle character(s) to be changed	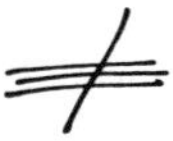 ⧸=
Change small capital letters to lower case letters	Encircle character(s) to be changed	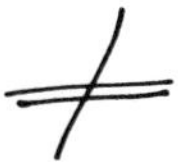 ⧸=
Change italic to upright type	Encircle character(s) to be changed	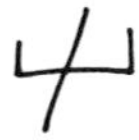 �

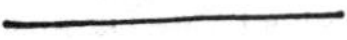

INSTRUCTION	TEXTUAL MARK	MARGINAL MARK
Invert type	Encircle character to be inverted	
Substitute or insert character in 'superior' position	/ through character or ⅄ where required	under character eg
Substitute or insert character in 'inferior' position	/ through character or ⅄ where required	over character eg
Substitute ligature eg fl for separate letters	⊢————⊣ through characters affected	eg fl
Substitute separate letters for ligature	⊢————⊣	Write out separate letters
Substitute or insert full stop or decimal point	/ through character or ⅄ where required	
Substitute or insert colon	/ through character or ⅄ where required	
Substitute or insert semi-colon	/ through character or ⅄ where required	;
Substitute or insert comma	/ through character or ⅄ where required	,

INSTRUCTION	TEXTUAL MARK		MARGINAL MARK
Substitute or insert apostrophe	/ or ⅄	through character / where required	〜
Substitute or insert single quotation marks	/ or ⅄	through character / where required	〜 and/or 〜
Substitute or insert double quotation marks	/ or ⅄	through character / where required	〜 and/or 〜
Substitute or insert ellipsis	/ or ⅄	through character / where required	• • •
Substitute or insert leader dots	/ or ⅄	through character / where required	(•••)
Substitute or insert hyphen	/ or ⅄	through character / where required	⊢
Substitute or insert rule	/ or ⅄	through character / where required	⊢
Substitute or insert oblique	/ or ⅄	through character / where required	(/)
Start new paragraph	⌐		⌐
Run on (no new paragraph)	⌇		⌇

INSTRUCTION	TEXTUAL MARK	MARGINAL MARK
Transpose characters or words	between characters or words, numbered where necessary	
Transpose a number of characters or words	3 2 1	123
Transpose lines		
Transpose a number of lines	3 2 1	
Centre	Enclosing matter to be centred	[ ]
Indent		
Cancel indent		
Set line justified to specified measure	and/or	
Set column justified to specified measure		
Move matter specified distance to the right	enclosing matter to be moved to the right	
Move matter specified distance to the left	enclosing matter to be moved to the left	

INSTRUCTION	TEXTUAL MARK	MARGINAL MARK
Take over character(s), word(s) or line to next line, column or page		
Take back character(s), word(s) or line to previous line, column or page		
Raise matter	over matter to be raised under matter to be raised	
Lower matter	over matter to be lowered under matter to be lowered	
Move matter to position indicated	Enclose matter to be moved and indicate new position	
Correct vertical alignment		
Correct horizontal alignment	Single line above and below misaligned matter eg misaligned	
Close up. Delete space between characters or words	Delete space	
Insert space between characters	between characters affected	
Insert space between words	between words affected	

INSTRUCTION	TEXTUAL MARK	MARGINAL MARK
Make space appear equal between characters or words	between characters or words affected	
Close up normal interline spacing	each side of column linking lines	
Insert space between lines or paragraphs	or	
Reduce space between lines or paragraphs	or	
Reduce space between characters	between characters affected	
Reduce space between words	between words affected	

Source : Barnard, *The Blueprint Handbook of Print and Production;* published by Chapman & Hall, 1994.

When your paper has been accepted 'the author may cite his forthcoming paper as "in press" and start thinking about the next one' (Smith, 1985: 168).

6.4 WRITING A LETTER TO A JOURNAL

> It is important to have something worthwhile to say. If you do not, then by all means write a letter, but don't post it.
>
> Calnan and Barabas (1973: 10)

Letters to the editor of a journal are an excellent way of sharing information or highlighting concerns with colleagues. In recent years the paramedical professions have begun to use this resource more widely, as appreciation of its value has grown. The main use of such letters are:

- to comment on an article published in the journal

- to advertise facilities or resources

- to indicate findings of a study which is not yet ready for publication

- to make 'controversial' statements.

Calnan and Barabas (1973: 8) cite the three common faults to avoid in writing a letter to a journal as 'pompous circumlocution about trivia, self-opinionated statements, and the lack of factual information'.

When writing a letter:

1. Address it 'Madam' (or 'Sir': remember to find out which is applicable).
2. Come to the point of the letter quickly. If you are commenting on a previous publication in the journal, provide the reference.
3. Wherever possible cite references to support your views. Do not make unsubstantiated statements. References should be given in full at the end of the letter (by convention the Harvard or Vancouver styles are used; see 6.2).
4. Be professional. If you are writing to disagree with a colleague, ensure that your criticisms are professional and constructive.
5. Finish 'Yours faithfully', sign your name, print your name, state your profession or qualifications if relevant and give an address.
6. Enclose a compliment slip confirming that the letter is for publication. (For example: 'I enclose a letter which I hope you will consider for publication.') You must specifically say if you do not want the letter edited. If you wish the letter to appear anonymously you should include sound reasons for this, although some editors find such letters unacceptable.

7. As a guide, remember that even the shortest letter has three paragraphs (Williams, 1989: 114). There must be an introduction to the subject matter, a point to be made and a conclusion or recommendation.

6.5   INSTRUCTIONS FOR TYPISTS

You only have to read a handful of dissertations or papers to see how generous authors are with thanks to their typists. Frequently these poor individuals are faced with inadequate instructions, poor handwriting and, to put it bluntly, deciphering rubbish. Nothing is ever obvious to someone else: it is not obvious that you wanted headings underlined twice or paragraphs indented unless you say so.

Always give your typist adequate instructions, preferably written down, which can be referred to. A telephone number where you can be reached can also be invaluable, particularly when you also have a copy of the work to be typed at hand.

Specific points

- Check around for an idea of the costs involved but remember that the cheapest may not be the best. Personal recommendation is a good guide to finding a good typist.

- If your handwriting is as bad as mine, make a concerted effort to be legible. Double spacing (writing on alternate lines) may make the task easier.

- Spell unusual medical/research terms carefully.

- If you need to make an insertion, label it carefully in the text. If there is more than one insertion, use letters or numbers to identify them, for example, insert A, insert B.

- Check the order of your pages; number them sequentially.

- Provide information on:
  - paper size
  - paper quality
  - margin size
  - spacing   • double or single
    - amount of space needed for diagrams
  - headings   • capitals or not
    - underlining or bold
  - layout   • new pages for each chapter/for each table
    - indented paragraphs.

When you receive your typed copy, proofread it carefully. Check punctuation, spelling (especially specialist terms), amount of space left for diagrams and the order of pages. Corrections are best done in coloured pen. You would also be well advised to ask one or two colleagues to check the proofs for you. They will be less familiar with the material than you are and so more likely to detect anomalies in content and typographical mistakes.

Always remember to consult the guidelines on presentation available from the university or journal to which you are submitting your work.

6.5.1 Using word processors

A basic word processor is more versatile than the most expensive and sophisticated typewriter, so even a novice can produce a professional looking document with only a few hours' practice. As most individuals now have access to a word processor, it is a good idea to become familiar with their use. Indeed, if you regularly pay to have work typed, it may be more astute to invest in a word processor and practise using it than to continue paying for secretarial services.

MacDonald (1984) noted that the main advantage of a word processor is that 'unlike even an experienced typist, it can never make new mistakes in the embedded text'. Layouts of documents can be experimented with and modifications made. Large sections of text can be moved around and additions made; mistakes can be corrected easily. New drafts can be produced quickly as you do not need to retype the whole document: all that is required is an update of the previous draft. Other features include spelling corrections, automatic page numbering and centring for headings. With some of the more up-market models you can leave the printer to print out the document while you do something else.

6.6 PREPARING A POSTER

Posters offer a relatively new method of sharing new research with colleagues at medical and scientific meetings. They are also becoming more widely used at paramedical study days and at conferences.

Points to consider

1. Visual attractiveness is vital. It is important to avoid overcrowding the poster with too much information, using too much (or indeed too little) colour or using too large (or too small) letters. Diagrams, graphs, pictures and photos can be used well in poster displays.

2. The poster should include:

- title (this should be succinct)
- author(s), professional address
- introduction, aims
- method(s)
- results (particularly tables and graphs)
- conclusions
- references (no more than five).

   The title should be written in the largest print with the names of the authors only slightly smaller. The rest of the text should be clear when standing a few feet away from the poster.
3. It is important to have details of the display stand so that you can practise the layout of the poster.
4. The presenter should carry scissors, sellotape, drawing pins or velcro mounts whenever you need to present a poster.
5. The author should be available at some point during the conference to answer questions on the project. It is useful to have handouts of information for delegates to take away.

6.7 PREPARING A TALK

   The tongue of the wise commends knowledge, but the mouth of the fool gushes folly.

   Proverbs 15, verse 2

Eminent researchers have ruined their reputations in minutes by speaking badly at meetings. We have all attended lectures and talks given by someone whose work we have admired, only to go away thinking that they had been greatly overrated. Talks are a valuable way of communicating research findings to others, but only if they are done properly. Public speaking is a skill. Consequently, like most skills, it does not come automatically. However, most people can learn to give a satisfactory talk providing they invest time and effort in preparing their material.

Points to note

1. A talk should have a beginning, a middle and an end.
2. Practise. Practise the talk, your timing and your delivery. Use a mirror, your friends and your colleagues. If at all possible, practise in the venue in which you will be speaking.
3. DO NOT READ YOUR TALK OUT. Most audiences can read so it would be easier to hand them out the text and let them read it themselves.

Use cue cards to help you. Remember: slides and other audiovisual aids are displayed behind you and should not be used as prompts.

4. Fully prepare all audiovisual materials.

5. Direct the talk towards your audience and amend your terminology as appropriate. Remember that the talk given to a League of Friends will be different from that given to a group of Physicians.

6. Stick to the title given. Present the talk you were asked to give and not the one you wanted to. It is amazing how frequently speakers drift off at a tangent from the talk they were actually asked to deliver.

7. Keep to a few simple themes. Do not try to present your entire research project in ten minutes.

8. Gain the attention of your audience quickly. How you do this is entirely up to you, but do not amble into a talk. State its aim immediately and set the scene.

9. Avoid complicated (usually boring) statistics. If you cannot explain your statistics simply, you do not understand them yourself.

10. Keep to time. It is rude to overrun your talk at the expense of other speakers and particularly the audience who will have other demands on their time.

11. Leave time for questions from the audience so that they have the opportunity of clarifying points you have made.

Your ability will be judged by the quality of the audiovisual aids you use, so ensure that they are good. Invest the money in getting the help of an expert, do not do it yourself. Familiarize yourself with the equipment you will need to use and ensure that your slides are in the correct order and the right way up. Make sure that the video is set to play the piece you need. Above all, do not flash up slides and say 'We won't bother with this.' If you are not going to show a slide for a reasonable time, do not present it at all. Take it out of the set before you begin.

It is a sad fact within the therapy professions that only a comparatively small number of therapists take time to read their professional journals. So talks give an important opportunity to communicate recent developments or problems to colleagues. On the other hand, the researcher who views talks as one-way traffic is making a huge mistake. Talks are an invaluable way to obtain feedback from others and receive comments at first hand. Important advice can be gained during and after talks from colleagues and contact can be made with people working in the same or similar fields.

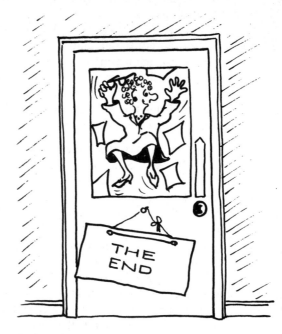

Figure 7.1 Conclusion.

With the end of the book virtually in sight, it seems appropriate to revisit the place where you and I began by noticing a parallel between the attributes of a good researcher and a good therapist. If we remind ourselves that, in Hockey's (1985) view, the ingredients of success in research are the curiosity, competence, integrity, common sense and sense of humour of the person carrying out the investigation, then it seems reasonable to wonder whether the preceding chapters have kindled your curiosity, hopefully with the occasional appeal to your sense of humour. Some sections of the text may have aroused your common sense; others may have been too packed with information for easy digestion. With any luck, you decided to reserve these for a later date, to be used as reference sections when you need to call on details of a range of research designs, tools of measurement or statistical analysis.

Beyond stating the obvious – that it has taken a goodly number of pages to cover our discussions on research methodology – can we draw any firm conclusions about the impact of these pages? At this stage, you as the reader might want to ask two questions: 'Why did you write the book?' and 'Have you achieved your purpose?' If you do **feel like asking** these questions, you are thinking in a research mode and part of the purpose of the book has been justified. My answer to your questions would have to be that the book was written with two interlocking aims: to interest therapists in becoming researchers and to promote a wider evaluation of health and social care. These aims converge to benefit our clients now and in the future, a) directly, by improvements to professional practice in response to research findings and by greater awareness on the part of the researcher and b) indirectly, by refining and adding to the knowledge base for the health professions. In itself this leads to increased competence on the part of their practitioners.

Instead of answering your questions, I might have countered a question with another question. I might have asked you: 'Have I interested you, as an individual, in the fascinating and challenging world of research, often at times frustrating but never dull?' If we review some of the **ideas** put forward among the **methods**, it might be easier for you, the reader, to give more than an unqualified 'NO' or 'YES' in answer to my question.

Research is timely in periods of resource scarcity. With escalating demands and limited resources, all health and social services are under pressure. There is widespread insistence on value for money and accountability to the consumer. This can only be met by regular and formal evaluation. In this climate of obligation to be effective and efficient, therapists who are interested in better systems for evaluating their services are likely to be encouraged rather than discouraged in setting up clear investigations. With a well-prepared proposal that addresses topical issues, there is every likelihood that funding will be found to allow the work to be carried out. Referring to the contribution of nurses and therapists to research and development in health services, Professor Adrian Webb said:

> There is an evident need to promote the development of a greater research capability within health services. This is particularly true for the two professional groups involved in this conference.
>
> Webb (1994: 37)

Research leads to more research. Once interest in research has been established and projects are completed and reported, the partial answers that are gained lead to more questions and highlight the need for continuing the process of evaluation and exploration. For example, if a study demonstrates that one stroke unit does better than another, the next question is: 'Why is this so?'

Research findings can change practice. Although not every published paper is immediately acclaimed, the real world of professional practice is influenced by research findings. Sometimes, recommendations arise from incidental discoveries, such as the value of a regular intake of aspirin in low doses for people who are at risk of myocardial infarction. In other cases, the results from research projects seem highly credible and the techniques recommended by the researchers have been quickly adopted.

Research encourages the establishment of research posts. Career opportunities are being opened up by the growing need for research. Managers who have targets for improving efficiency and for finding the best use of manpower are under pressure to commission evaluation studies so that evidence of good practice can be gathered. In the words of Professor Webb:

> There is also a need to develop a culture in which managers, in commissioning authorities and in provider units, can support the ideas that nurses and therapists, as well as other health care professionals, contribute to all levels of research and development activities.
>
> Webb (1994)

In tandem with this need, all the health professions are developing standards of practice to be used in their regular auditing of services. These pressures are being met by the establishment of research posts; some of these are multidisciplinary while others are offered within a speciality. As a result the priority for research funding within annual budgets has risen. Speaking at a national conference, Professor John Marshall of the Stroke Association gave his support for this change in priorities by commenting that:

> Those who say money spent on research would be better spent on helping patients tend to forget that today's treatment was yesterday's research.
>
> Marshall (1995)

Research standards should be consistently high. Remember that reputations, your own and that of your colleagues, rest on the quality of your studies. It is important to 'stick to the rules' and to ensure that no bad or unethical procedures are condoned by you or your assistant researchers.

Research results need to be shared. The work of completing a research study is never over until one or more papers have been written for publication. This is one way of making sure that your results can be considered and debated by your colleagues on a national or even an international basis. Never be discouraged if your published work attracts some criticism. This can give you the advantage of continuing a discussion and of learning with and from your critics. It is far better to attract critical or advisory comments than to have no feedback at all. And it is worth noting that research reports are often welcomed by people working in your field of interest.

Once the work has been written up, there are likely to be opportunities to present your findings at conferences and professional meetings. Remember that these include spoken and poster presentations: all these give you the opportunity to exchange ideas with your colleagues and to recharge your personal reserve of enthusiasm. Perhaps the most rewarding part of joining the people who are committed to research is the excitement of finding that other people want to hear your opinions, sharpen their ideas by trying them on you and treat your questions with keen interest.

You will never know the pleasures (or woes) of research until you try them.

References

Adkins, D. (1974) 2nd edn *Test Construction: Development and Interpretation of Achievement Test*, Merrill, Columbus.

Adorno, T.W. (1950) *The Authoritarian Personality*, Harper & Row, New York.

Albert, M.L. (1973) A simple test of visual neglect. *Neurology*, **23**, 658–64.

Allen, E.M. (1960) Why are research grant applications disapproved? *Science*, **132**, 1532–4.

Altman, D.G. (1982) How large a sample? in Gore, S.M. and Altman, D.G. *Statistics in Practice*, British Medical Association, London, pp. 6–8.

Anderson, B., Llewellyn, G. and Bell, J. (1991) Records: one measure of occupational therapy practice in the field of development disabilities. *Australian Journal of Occupational Therapy*, **38** (2), 77–81.

Apley, J. (1976) Pleasures of medical writing. *British Medical Journal*, **1**, 999–1001.

Barber, A.S., Barraclough, E.D. and Gray, W.A. (1972) Closing the gap between the medical researcher and the literature. *British Medical Journal*, **1**, 368–70.

Barlow, D.H. and Hersen, M. (1984) *Single Case Experimental Designs*, Pergamon Press, Oxford.

Barton, A.H. (1958) Asking the embarrassing question. *Public Opinion Quarterly*, **22**, 67–8.

Bausell, R.B. (1986) *A Practical Guide to Conducting Empirical Research*, Harper & Row, London, pp. 44–51.

Beard, D.J. and Fergusson, C.M. (1992) The conservative management of anterior cruciate ligament deficiency. A nationwide survey of current practice. *Physiotherapy*, **78** (3), 181–5.

Bennett, A.E. and Ritchie, K. (1975) *Questionnaires in Medicine: a Guide to their Design and Use*, Oxford University Press, London, pp. 6–7.

Blowman, C., Pickles, C., Emery, S., Creates, V., Towell, L., Blackburn, N., Doyle, N. and Walkden, B. (1991) Prospective double blind controlled trial of intensive physiotherapy with and without stimulation of the pelvic floor in treatment of genuine stress incontinence. *Physiotherapy*, **77** (10), 661–4.

Bourke, G.J. and McGilvray, J. (1975) 2nd edn *Interpretation and Uses of Medical Statistics*, Blackwell Scientific Publications, Oxford, pp. 131–5.

Boyle, C.M. (1970) Difference between patients' and doctors' interpretation of some common medical terms. *British Medical Journal*, **2**, 286–9.

Bradford-Hill, A. (1965) The reason for writing. *British Medical Journal*, **2**, 870.

Breakwell, G.M. (1990) *Problems in Practice: Interviewing*, British Psychological Society and Routledge, Leicester and London.

British Medical Association (BMA) (1971) *Research Funds Guide*, BMA Planning Unit, London.

British Medical Association (BMA) (1987) *Medical Libraries: a User's Guide*, BMA Professional and Scientific Division, London.

Bryman, A. (1989) *Research Methods and Organizational Studies*, Unwin Hyman, London.

Burns, N. and Grove, S.K. (1987) *The Practice of Nursing Research: Conduct, Critique and Utilization*, Saunders, Philadelphia.

Burl, M.M., Williams, J.G. and Nayak, U.S.L. (1992) The effect of cervical collars on walking balance. *Physiotherapy*, **78** (1), 19–22.

Calnan, J. (1976) *One Way to Do Research: The A–Z for Those who Must*, Heinemann, London.

Calnan, J. (1984) *Coping with Research: the Complete Guide for Beginners*, Heinemann Medical, London.

Calnan, J. and Barabas, A. (1973) *Writing Medical Papers: a Practical Guide*, Heinemann, London.

Carr, E.K. (1991) Observational methods in rehabilitation research. *Clinical Rehabilitation*, **5**, 89–94.

Castle, W.M. (1977) 2nd edn *Statistics in Small Doses*, Churchill Livingstone, London.

Cheng, S. and Rogers, J.C. (1989) Changes in occupational role performance after a severe burn: a retrospective study. *American Journal of Occupational Therapy*, **43** (1), 17–24.

Chenitz, W.C. and Swanson, J.M. (1986) *From Practice to Grounded Theory: Qualitative Research in Nursing*, Addison Wesley, Menlo Park, California.

Cohen, J. (1977) *Statistical Power Analysis for the Behavioural Sciences*, Academic Press, New York.

Collin, C., Wade, D.T., Davis, S. and Horne, V. (1988) The Barthel ADL index: a reliability study. *International Disability Studies*, **10**, 61–3.

Connolly, M.J., Wilkinson, E., Flanagan, S. and Mulley, G.P. (1990) Nurses' attitudes to and use of patient hoists in hospital. *Clinical Rehabilitation*, **4**, 13–17.

Cooke, D.J. (1989) *Epidemiological and Mental Health Research: a Handbook of Skills and Methods*, Lawrence Erlbaum Associates, Hove/London, pp. 291–4.

Copyright, Designs and Patents Act (1988) HMSO, London.

Cormack, D.F.S. (ed.) (1984) *The Research Process in Nursing*, Blackwell Scientific, Oxford.

Currier, D.P. (1984) *Elements of Research in Physical Therapy*, Williams & Wilkins, Baltimore.

Data Protection Act (1984) HMSO, London.

Disraeli, B. (1804–81) in Andrews, R. (1993) *The Columbia Dictionary of Quotations*, Columbia University Press, New York, p. 870.

Drummond, A.E.R. (1990) Symposium on methodology. *Surveys, Clinical Rehabilitation*, **4**, 255–9.

Drummond, A.E.R. and Walker, M.F. (1995) A randomised controlled trial of leisure rehabilitation after stroke. *Clinical Rehabilitation*, **9**, 283–90.

Edwards, A. (1957) *Techniques of Attitude Scale Construction*, Appleton-Century-Crofts, New York.

Elman, S.A. (1975) Cost comparison of manual and on-line computerised literature searching. *Special Libraries*, **66** (1), 12–18.

Evans, K.M. (1978) *Planning Small Scale Research*, NFER-Nelson, Windsor.

Fowkes, F.G.R. and Fulton, P.M. (1991) Critical appraisal of published research: Introduction guidelines. *British Medical Journal*, **302**, 1136–40.

Gee, H. (1991) Effects of group treatment on interpersonal behaviour of elderly clients with dementia. *Australian Journal of Occupational Therapy*, **38** (2), 63–7.

Gold, R.L. (1958) Roles in sociological field observations. *Social Forces*, **36**, 217–23.

Goldstone, L.A. (1983) *Understanding Medical Statistics*, Heinemann Medical Books, London.

Gore, S.M. (1981) Assessing clinical trials: trial size. *British Medical Journal*, **282**, 1687–9.

Greene, J. and d'Oliveira, M. (1981) *Methodology Handbook*, Open University, Milton Keynes.

Gunning, R. (1968) *The Technique of Clear Writing*, McGraw Hill, New York.

Hamburger, J. (1968) Some general considerations, in Wolstenholme, G. and O'Connor, M. (eds) *Law and Ethics of Transplantation*, CIBA Foundation Blueprints, J & A Churchill, London, pp. 134–48.

Hicks, C.M. (1988) *Practical Research Methods for Physiotherapists*, Churchill Livingstone, London.

Hilgard, E.R., Atkinson, R.L. and Atkinson, R.C. (1979) 7th edn *Introduction to Psychology*, Harcourt Brace Jovanovich, New York.

Hockey, L. (1985) *Nursing Research: Mistakes and Misconceptions*, Churchill Livingstone, London.

House of Lords Select Committee on Science and Technology. Session 1987–1988, *Priorities in Medical Research*, 3rd Report, HMSO, London, paras. 3.1 and 3.2.

Howie, J. (1978) Applying for a research grant. *British Medical Journal*, **2**, 1553–4.

Huff, D. (1954) *How to Lie with Statistics*, Penguin Books, Harmondsworth.

Huth, E.J. (1982) How to write and publish papers in the medical sciences, in Hawkins, C. and Sorgi, M. (eds) (1985) *Research. How to Plan, Speak and Write About It*, Springer-Verlag, Berlin.

International Committee of Medical Journal Editors (1982) Uniform requirements of manuscripts submitted to biomedical journals. *British Medical Journal*, **284**, 1766–70.

Jenkins, S.R. (1985) Searching the literature, in Hawkins, C. and Sorgi, M. (eds) *Research. How to Plan, Speak and Write About It*, Springer-Verlag, Berlin.

Jolley, J. (1991) Computing in practice: Using statistics. *Nursing Times*, 19 June, **87** (25), 57–9.

Jones, A. (1990) *How to Write a Winning CV*, Hutchinson Business Books, London.

Juby, L.C., Lincoln, N.B. and Berman, P. (1996) The effect of a stroke rehabilitation unit on functional and psychological outcome: a randomised control trial. *Cerebrovascular Diseases*, **6**, 106–10.

Kane, E. (1985) *Doing Your Own Research*, Marion Boyars, London.

Kaye, S. (1991) The value of audit in clinical practice. *Physiotherapy*, **77** (10), 705–7.

Kerlinger, F.N. (1986) *Foundations of Behavioural Research*, Holt, Rienhart & Winston, New York.

Kirkwood, B.R. (1988) *Essentials of Medical Statistics*, Blackwell Scientific, Oxford.

Lincoln, N.B. (1990) Research methodology. *Clinical Rehabilitation*, **4**, 91–3.

LoBiondo-Wood, G. and Haber, J. (1990) *Nursing Research. Methods, Critical Appraisal and Utilization*, Mosby, Saint Louis.

MacDonald, P. (1984) Writing a thesis on a word processor. *British Medical Journal*, **289**, 242–3.

Mahoney, F.I. and Barthel, D.W. (1965) Functional evaluation: the Bartherl Index. *Maryland State Medical Journal*, **14**, 61–5.

Makrides, L. and Richman, J. (1981) Research methodology and applied statistics. Part 6: Ethics in human research. *Physiotherapy Canada*, **33** (2), 89–94.

Marshall, J. (1995) Report of The Stroke Association's National Fieldstaff Conference. *Stroke News*, **13** (2), 4.

McGuire, B.E. and Greenwood, R.J. (1990) Effects of an intervention aimed at memory on perceived burden and self-esteem after traumatic head injury. *Clinical Rehabilitation*, **4**, 319–23.

Merritt, D.H. (1963) Grantmanship: an exercise in lucid presentation. *Clinical Research*, **11**, 375–7.

Miller, P. McC. and Wilson, M.J. (1983) *A Dictionary of Social Science Methods*, Wiley, Chichester.

Moffett, A.K. (1991) Randomised controlled trials. *Clinical Rehabilitation*, **5**, 1–4.

Nouri, F.M. and Lincoln, N.B. (1987) An extended activities of daily living scale for stroke patients. *Clinical Rehabilitation*, **1**, 301–5.

O'Brien, E. (1990) Prepare a curriculum vitae, in *How To Do It*, Vol. 1, BMJ Publishing Group, London, pp. 149–55.

Ogier, M. (1989) *Reading Research: How to Make Research More Approachable*, Scutari, London.

Oppenheim, A. (1966) *Questionnaire Design and Attitude Measurement*, Heinemann, London.

Parahoo, K. and Reid, N. (1988) Critical reading of research. *Nursing Times*, 26 October, **84** (43), 69–72.

Partridge, C. and Barnitt, R. (1986) *Research Guidelines: a Handbook for Therapists*, Heinemann, London.

Pentlelow, G.M. (1989) New technology in medical libraries. *British Medical Journal*, **298**, 907–8.

Reid, D.T. (1992) A survey of Canadian occupational therapists' use of hand splints for children with neuromuscular dysfunction. *Canadian Journal of Occupational Therapy*, **59** (1), 16–27.

Reid, D. and Drake, S. (1990) A comparative study of visual perceptual skills in normal children and children with diplegic cerebral palsy. *Canadian Journal of Occupational Therapy*, **57** (3), 141–6.

Reid, N.G. and Boore, J.R.P. (1987) *Research Methods and Statistics in Health Care*, Edward Arnold, London.

Richardson, A., Jackson, C. and Sykes, W. (1990) *Taking Research Seriously*, HMSO, London.

Roberts, D. (1990) Index Medicus and Medline for occupational therapists. Part 1: An overview of coverage and searching methods. *British Journal of Occupational Therapy*, **53** (8), 317–20.

Roberts, N.A. (1990) Prospective follow-up study of elderly patients discharged from an accident and emergency department. *Clinical Rehabilitation*, **4**, 37–41.

Robinson, V.M. (1977) *Humor and the Health Professions*, Slack Inc, New Jersey, p. 160.

Rowntree, D. (1981) *Statistics Without Tears: A Primer for Non-mathematicians*, Penguin Books, Harmondsworth.

Royal College of Physicians (1986) *Research on Healthy Volunteers*, Royal College of Physicians, London.

Royal College of Physicians (1990) *Research Involving Patients*, January, Royal College of Physicians, London.

Sackett, D.L. (1979) Bias in analytical research. *Journal of Chronic Disability*, **32**, 51–63.

Sax, G. (1980) 2nd edn *Principles of Educational and Psychological Measurement and Evaluation*, Wadsworth, Belmont, California.

Seaman, C.H.C. (1987) 3rd edn *Research Methods: Principles, Practice and Theory for Nursing*, Appleton and Lange, Connecticut.

Shinar, D., Gross, C.R., Bronstein, K.S., Licata-Gehr, E.E., Eden, D.T. *et al.* (1987) Reliability of the activities of daily living scale and its use in telephone interview. *Archives of Medical Rehabilitation*, **68**, 723–8.

Shott, S. (1990) *Statistics for Health Professionals*, Saunders, Philadelphia.

Siegel, S. and Castellan, N.J. (1988) *Non-parametric Systems for the Behavioural Sciences*, McGraw-Hill, New York.

Simon, J.L. (1969) *Basic Research Methods in Social Science*, Random House Inc., New York, pp. 97–8.

Smith, J. (1985) Publication, Chapter 8, in Hawkins, C. and Sorgi, M. (eds) *Research. How to Plan, Speak and Write About It*, Springer-Verlag, Berlin, pp. 153–69.

Smith, R. (1991) Your article: what happens to it? *Australian Occupational Therapy Journal*, **39** (2), 107.

Spry, V.M., Hovell, M.F., Sallis, J.G., Hopsetter, C.R., Elder, J.P. and Molgaard, C.A. (1989) Recruiting survey respondents to mailed surveys: controlled trials of incentives and prompts. *American Journal of Epidemiology*, **130**, 166–72.

Sternberg, R.J. (1988) 2nd edn *The Psychologist's Companion. A Guide to Scientific Writing for Students and Researchers*, Cambridge University Press, Cambridge.

Sunderland, A. (1990) Single-case experiments in neurological rehabilitation. *Clinical Rehabilitation*, **4**, 181–92.

Sutcliffe, P. (1992) The occupational therapy labour market. Part 1: making use of trained personnel. *British Journal of Occupational Therapy*, **55** (1), 13–18.

Sylvester, K.L. (1990) Investigation of the effect of hydrotherapy in the treatment of osteoarthritic hips. *Clinical Rehabilitation*, **4** (3), 223–8.

Temple, M. (1978) *Get it Right! A Pocket Guide to Written English*, John Murray, London.

Thurstone, L. and Chave, E. (1929) *The Measurement of Attitude*, University of Chicago Press, Chicago.

Timbury, M.C. (1979) How to do it: use a library. *British Medical Journal*, **1**, 252–3.

Treece, E.W. and Treece, J.W. (1977) 2nd edn *Elements of Research in Nursing*, Mosby, Saint Louis.

Wainwright, G. (1984) *Report Writing*, Management Update, London.

Wartenberg, D. and Greenberg, M. (1990) Detecting disease clusters: the importance of statistical power. *American Journal of Epidemiology*, (supplement 1), S1, 56–66.

Webb, A. (1994) *The Nursing and Therapy Professions' Contribution to Health Services Research and Development*, conference report, 12 May 1994, Department of Health.

Weisberg, H.F. and Bowen, B.D. (1977) *An Introduction to Survey Research and Data Analysis*, Freeman, San Francisco.

Whiting, S.E., Lincoln, N.B., Bhavnani, G. and Cockburn, J. (1985) *The Rivermead Perceptual Assessment Battery*, NFER-Nelson, Windsor.

Williams, K. (1989) *Study Skills*, Macmillan Professional Masters, London.

Wilson, S.L., Cranny, S.M. and Andrews, K. (1992) The efficacy of music stimulation in prolonged coma: four single case experiments. *Clinical Rehabilitation*, **6** (3), 181–7.

Working for patients (1989) Department of Health, p. 38, para. 4.30.

World Medical Association (1964) Declaration of Helsinki. *British Medical Journal*, **2**, 177.

Wright, G. and Fowler, C. (1986) *Investigative Design and Statistics*, Penguin Books, Harmondsworth.

Index